TREATING EXPLOSIVE KIDS

Treating Explosive Kids

The Collaborative Problem-Solving Approach

ROSS W. GREENE
J. STUART ABLON

THE GUILFORD PRESS
NEW YORK   LONDON

© 2006 Ross W. Greene and J. Stuart Ablon; revisions for third printing © 2006
Published by The Guilford Press
A Division of Guilford Publications, Inc.
370 Seventh Avenue, Suite 1200, New York, NY 10001
www.guilford.com

Printed in the United States of America

This book is printed on acid-free paper.

Last digit is print number: 9

Library of Congress Cataloging-in-Publication Data

Greene, Ross W.
   Treating explosive kids : the collaborative problem-solving approach /
Ross W. Greene, J. Stuart Ablon.
       p. cm.
Includes bibliographical references and index.
ISBN-10: 1-59385-203-7   ISBN-13: 978-1-59385-203-0 (cloth)
   1.   Problem children.   2.   Behavior disorders in children.   3.   Child
rearing.   4.   Parent and child.   I. Ablon, J. Stuart.   II. Title.
   HQ773.G737 2006
   649.'153—dc22   2005010758

If I am not for myself, who is for me?
If I am only for myself, what am I?
If not now, when?
—HILLEL

Illusions are the truths we live by
until we know better.
—NANCY GIBBS

About the Authors

Ross W. Greene, PhD, is founder and director of *Lives in the Balance* and the originator of the Collaborative & Proactive Solutions approach, as described in his books *The Explosive Child* and *Lost at School*. He is also adjunct Associate Professor in the Department of Psychology at Virginia Tech. In addition to providing outpatient care, he consults to schools, inpatient units, and residential and juvenile detention facilities. Dr. Greene's research focuses on the classification and treatment of explosive children; long-term outcomes in socially impaired children with attention-deficit/hyperactivity disorder (ADHD); and the impact of teacher characteristics on school outcome for elementary school students with ADHD. He has written extensively on behavioral assessment and social functioning; school- and home-based interventions for children with disruptive behavior disorders; and student–teacher compatibility. His research has been funded by the Stanley Medical Research Institute, the National Institute on Drug Abuse, and the U.S. Department of Education. Dr. Greene received his doctorate in clinical psychology from Virginia Tech after completing his predoctoral internship at Children's National Medical Center/George Washington University Medical Center in Washington, DC.

J. Stuart Ablon, PhD, is the Director of Think:Kids in the Department of Psychiatry at Massachusetts General Hospital where he specializes in the treatment of explosive children and adolescents and their families. He is also Associate Clinical Professor of Psychology in the Department of Psychiatry at Harvard Medical School. He consults extensively to schools, inpatient units, and residential and juvenile detention facilities. Dr. Ablon's research focuses on the process and outcome of psychosocial interventions, particularly the treatment of explosive children. He has authored numerous articles, chapters, and scientific papers on behavioral assessment and psychosocial interventions for children with disruptive behavior disorders. Dr. Ablon's research has been funded by the National Institutes of Health, the American Psychological Association, the Mood and Anxiety Disorders Institute, and the Endowment for the Advancement of Psychotherapy. Dr. Ablon received his doctorate in clinical psychology from the University of California at Berkeley and completed his pre- and postdoctoral training at Massachusetts General Hospital and Harvard Medical School.

Acknowledgments

We gratefully acknowledge our editor, Kitty Moore, for her patience in dealing with two obsessive authors who took some liberties with the "deadline" concept, and our agent, Wendy Lipkind, for her friendship and continued faith in our work. We also want to thank Tom Ollendick, Richard Johansson, Kim Bortle, Vance Heaney, and Michael Allan for their thoughtful comments on early drafts of the book, and Sarah Rabbitt for her assistance with the manuscript and for holding down the fort so we could write.

We would like to acknowledge those whose work directly or indirectly influenced our thinking. For RWG, this includes my mentor, Tom Ollendick; two extraordinary clinical supervisors, George Clum and Mary Ann McCabe; the person who got me interested in psychology in the first place, Betsy Altmaier; and a remarkable social worker named Lorraine Lougee, who taught me something about where the buck stops. And I want to dedicate the book to the memory of my grandmother, Clara Snider. Never one to mince words, she made the following astute observation of the CPS model: "It sounds like a lot of work."

For JSA, this includes a phenomenal researcher and clinician, Stephen Hinshaw; a clinical supervisor and parent who could not be more intuitive, Bonnie Ohye; and two extremely talented clinicians who also happen to be my parents. Finally, I would like to dedicate this book to my lifelong mentor in the study of human behavior, my grandfather, who frequently reminds me that we'd all be a lot better off if we did more thinking than feeling.

Contents

Chapter 1

Explosive Children and Adolescents

The Need for a Different Paradigm

Many labels have been used to describe the children and adolescents who are the focus of this book: defiant, aggressive, angry, raging, intransigent, resistant, willful, noncompliant, challenging, to name but a few. They've also been given disparate diagnoses, including oppositional defiant disorder (ODD), conduct disorder (CD), "conduct problems," and intermittent explosive disorder. Regardless of label, these youth present the most common (and among the most challenging) of referral problems to outpatient, inpatient, residential, juvenile detention, and school-based clinicians. Paradoxically, they are among the most poorly understood child and adolescent clinical populations.

We will use the term "explosive" to refer to these children and adolescents (for ease of exposition, we'll just call them "children" or "kids" henceforth) because we think this terminology best captures the behaviors causing upheaval, instability, and frustration in these children and in their adult caretakers, namely, severe resistance to the imposition of adult will and corresponding explosive outbursts. As one might expect, research has shown these characteristics to have extremely deleterious effects on interactions between the children who exhibit them and their adult caretakers (e.g., Anastopoulos, Guevremont, Shelton, & DuPaul, 1992; Arnold & O'Leary, 1995; Barkley, Anastopoulos, Guevremont, & Fletcher, 1992; Greene, Beszterczey, Katzenstein, Park, & Goring, 2002; Greene, Biederman, et al., 2002; Stormschak, Speltz, DeKlyen, & Greenberg, 1997; see Lytton, 1990). We do not make a major distinction between the less serious forms of these characteristics that might lead to a diagnosis of ODD and the more serious forms that might lead to a diagnosis of CD. We have found that explosive children are helped by the model of care described in this book irrespective of the diagnoses used to capture their difficulties.

Of course, neither "explosive" nor any other label captures the complex array of difficulties frequently seen in these children. This leads to some very important themes that are woven throughout the whole of this text:

1. *Explosive children are a heterogeneous group.*
2. *One's understanding of the factors underlying a specific child's explosive behaviors directly influences the selection of interventions employed to address those behaviors.*
3. *There is no "one size fits all approach" to the treatment of explosive children and their adult caretakers.*
4. *Intervention options are most potent when they are well matched to the needs of those persons for whom intervention is being designed.*

The model of care described in this book—*Collaborative Problem Solving (CPS)*—embodies these themes and springs from the awareness that the difficulties of explosive children are not only poorly understood, but, in many instances, also poorly addressed by available therapies. Historically, what types of interventions have been applied to this population of children? For approximately the past 45 years, conceptualization and treatment of explosive behavior have been strongly influenced by the coercion, or social interactional, model (e.g., Hanf, 1970; Patterson & Gullion, 1968; Patterson, Reid, & Dishion, 1992; see Taylor & Biglan, 1998). Indeed, this well-disseminated model has become the standard of care for youth with disruptive behavior disorders.

While there is no singular coercion theory, most representations of the model have focused primarily on patterns of parental discipline that contribute to the development of coercive parent–child exchanges. For example, as described by Chamberlain and Patterson (1995), four subtypes of "parent inadequate discipline" have been identified, including *inconsistent discipline*

(parents who respond indiscriminately to a child's positive and negative behaviors, evidence poor or inconsistent follow-through with commands, give in
when a child argues, and unpredictably change expectations and consequences for rule violations); *irritable explosive discipline* (parents who issue
high rates of direct commands, frequently use high-intensity, high-amplitude
strategies such as hitting, yelling, and threatening, and frequently make humiliating or negative statements about the child); *low supervision and involvement* (parents who are unaware of their child's activities outside of their direct
supervision, do not know with whom the child is associating, are unaware of
their child's adjustment at school, rarely engage in joint activities with the
child, and are unwilling or unable to provide supervision even when aware of
the child's association with antisocial peers), and *inflexible rigid discipline*
(parents who rely on a single or limited range of discipline strategies for all
types of transgressions, fail to take contextual or extenuating factors into account, consistently fail to provide rationales or to use other induction tech-
niques in the context of discipline confrontations, and fail to adjust the intensity of the discipline reaction to the severity of the child's infraction). It is
these patterns of inadequate discipline, it is said, that contribute to a pattern of
adult–child interactions in which the child learns that arguing and tantrums
are an effective means of coercing adults into capitulating to his or her wishes.

The coercion model provides an excellent example of the manner by
which one's understanding of the factors underlying a child's explosive behaviors directly influences the interventions selected to address those behaviors.
If one perceives these behaviors to be the by-product of inconsistent, non-
contingent disciplinary practices, then the goal of intervention is self-evident:
teach adults to be more consistent and more contingent so as to help the child
learn that his or her arguing and tantrums will not coerce the adults into capitulating. Many variants of this approach exist, most subsumed under the general category of "parent management training," or PMT. The tools of this influ-
ential approach are familiar: (1) establish a list of target behaviors, with
compliance with adult directives as the primary objective; (2) establish a menu
of rewards and punishments, so as to give the child the incentive to comply
with adult directives; and (3) develop a currency system—points, stickers, to-
kens, levels, and the like—so as to track the child's performance and trigger
the dispensing of rewards and punishments.

An impressive body of research has documented the efficacy of PMT, and
is sufficiently compelling to qualify PMT as an empirically supported, well-
established treatment (e.g., Alexander & Parsons, 1973; Bernal, Klinnert, &
Schultz, 1980; Webster-Stratton, 1984, 1990, 1994; Wiltz & Patterson, 1974;
see Brestan & Eyberg, 1998; also see Pelham, Wheeler, & Chronis, 1998).

However, research has also documented various limitations of PMT (see Cavell, 2000). First, a substantial number of parents who receive PMT do not fully comply with implementation or drop out of treatment altogether (e.g., Prinz & Miller, 1994), suggesting that this form of intervention may not be well matched to the needs and characteristics of many of those responsible for implementation. Most studies examining the efficacy of PMT have presented data only for those who *remained* in treatment rather than for those who *began* treatment. Among parents who remain in treatment, PMT has been shown to produce statistically significant changes in oppositional behavior, but very few studies have reported clinically significant changes (Kazdin, 1997). Indeed, 30–40% of such parents continue to report child behavior problems in the clinical range at follow-up (e.g., Kazdin, 1993; Webster-Stratton, 1990). Data have shown that a significant percentage of children—perhaps higher than 50%—are not functioning within the normal range when such treatment is terminated (Dishion & Patterson, 1992). Finally, most studies examining the efficacy of PMT have not included clinically referred youth (Kazdin, 1997; Patterson & Chamberlain, 1994), and have typically failed to examine long-term treatment effects (Kazdin, 1993, 1997), although noteworthy exceptions to the latter issue exist (e.g., Ialongo et al., 1993). In view of these limitations, it is reasonable to conclude the following about PMT: (1) a meaningful percentage of children and parents do not derive substantial benefit from this model of intervention, and therefore (2) alternative treatments that more adequately address the needs of these children and their adult caretakers must be developed and studied. We believe that the limitations of PMT can be best understood—and the impetus for developing alternative treatments best found—in developmental theories that emphasize the transactional/reciprocal nature of interactions between children and adults.

TRANSACTIONAL THEORY

Sameroff (1975) has described three conceptual models for understanding children's developmental outcomes. The first—called the "unidirectional or main effect model"—proposes that a child's outcome is the product of *either* characteristics of the child *or* characteristics of his adult caretakers. From a unidirectional perspective, the following might be invoked to "explain" a child's explosive behavior (note that we'll be using the masculine gender throughout much of the remainder of the book): "He's explosive and noncompliant because his parents are inept disciplinarians" (here the characteristics of the parents are used to explain the child's maladaptive behavior) or "He's explosive and noncompliant because he has ADHD [attention-deficit/hyperactivity disorder]" (here characteristics of the child are invoked to explain the child's maladaptive behavior). Because such a model focuses on only one element of the adult–child equation, it greatly narrows the range of intervention options one might consider. Indeed, such a perspective gives rise to only two potential therapeutic options: (1) fix the problem adult or (2) fix the problem child.

The second model—called the "bidirectional or interactional model"—posits that it is the *combination* of adult and child characteristics that produces a child's outcome. This is a step in the right direction, for it includes both dimensions of the adult–child equation and therefore greatly expands the range of intervention options one might logically apply. However, this model treats outcome as something of a mathematics equation, whereby the combination of "good" child and adult characteristics produces a "good" outcome, the combination of "bad" child and adult characteristics produces a "bad" outcome, and combinations of "good" and "bad" produce "medium" outcomes. Such mathematics equations, of course, cannot account for those circumstances in which the combination of "good" adult characteristics and "good" child characteristics produce "bad" outcomes, or scenarios where the combination of "bad" adult characteristics and "bad" child characteristics produce "good" outcomes.

The third model—called the "transactional or reciprocal model"—posits that a child's outcome is a function of the degree of "fit" or "compatibility" between child and adult characteristics. A high degree of adult–child compatibility is thought to produce optimal outcomes, whereas a high level of incompatibility is thought to produce less optimal outcomes. From a transactional perspective, explosive behavior would simply be viewed as *one of many possible manifestations of adult–child incompatibility*, in which the characteristics of one interaction partner (e.g., the child) are poorly matched to the characteristics of the second interaction partner (e.g., the adult), thereby contributing to disadvantageous behavior in both partners and, over time, to more durable patterns of incompatibility. Other manifestations of adult–child incompatibility might include (but would by no means be limited to) child maltreatment, anxiety (in child or adult), depressed mood (in child or adult), social withdrawal (in child or adult), or abuse of substances (in child or adult) (e.g., Belsky, 1980; Cicchetti & Lynch, 1993, 1995). The transactional model clearly sets the stage for a departure from "fix the problem child" and "fix the problem adult" models of intervention. From a transactional perspective, the goal of treatment is to *improve compatibility between child and adult*. Such a goal requires an understanding of the characteristics of both *child and adult* and the involvement of both *child and adult* in whatever form of treatment is applied.

Is the coercion model transactional? Certainly the model has evolved from placing almost exclusive emphasis on inept parenting practices as the major determinant of childhood conduct problems (e.g., Patterson, DeBaryshe, & Ramsey, 1989) to an acknowledgment that child characteristics may also contribute to the development of maladaptive adult–child interactions (e.g., Dishion, French, & Patterson, 1995; Patterson et al., 1992). This evolution has presumably been prompted by compelling data underscoring the transactional, reciprocal nature of adult–child interactions (e.g., Anderson, Lytton, & Romney, 1986; Dumas & LaFreniere, 1993; Dumas, LaFreniere, & Serketich, 1995). However, for a model of development to be considered transactional, it must explain how child and adult, in combination with environmental factors, *influence each other and shape the course of each other's development* (e.g., Bell, 1968; Belsky, 1984; Chess & Thomas, 1984; Cicchetti & Lynch, 1993, 1995; Gottlieb, 1992; Sameroff, 1975, 1995). Whether current representations of coercion theory offer such an explanation is worthy of brief examination.

The fact that a coercive cycle requires two interaction partners does not, in and of itself, confer transactional status. As suggested by the patterns of parent inadequate discipline described above, the coercion model still places primary emphasis on parental characteristics rather than on reciprocal influences. Especially lacking is an elucidation of the manner by which specific *child* characteristics may contribute to the development of explosive behavior and the manner by which treatment plans would take such characteristics into account. Indeed, most recent representations of the coercion model do not view child characteristics as a necessary consideration in the development of coercive cycles, though it is quite clear that inept or inadequate parenting practices are viewed as essential to the development of such cycles (e.g., Dishion et al., 1995; Patterson et al., 1992; Snyder, Edwards, McGraw, Kilgore, & Holton, 1994). Further, coercion theory appears to view the coercive cycle as the sole factor contributing to explosive and noncompliant behavior in children. As noted above, from a transactional perspective, myriad manifestations of adult–child incompatibility might contribute to the development of explosive behavior. The historical overemphasis on adult characteristics in the development of explosive and noncompliant behavior has contributed to an underemphasis on the other "player" influencing adult–child compatibility: *the child*. Shirk (e.g., 2001) has argued that the "developmental invariance myth"—the belief that identical pathogenic mechanisms underlie the difficulties of all children with the same disorder—has been applied to many childhood psychiatric disorders. We believe this certainly has been the case with explosive behavior. To truly capture the transactional processes setting the stage for this behavior requires closer examination of child characteristics that also influence adult–child incompatibility.

In reviewing these child characteristics, *it is not our goal to establish the primacy of child characteristics in the development of explosive behavior.* Rather, we wish to emphasize the importance and implications of taking such characteristics into account in a transactional conceptualization of this behavior. Clearly, children's behavior does not develop independently of adult teaching and modeling (Kochanska, 1993). Nor do children's capacities for complying with adult directives develop independently of the manner by which caregivers impose expectations for compliance and respond to deviations from these expectations. Indeed, the method by which caregivers respond to such deviations can alter or fuel emerging response biases in both child and adult (e.g., Hoffman, 1983; Kochanska & Askan, 1995; Kopp, 1989).

CHILD CHARACTERISTICS ASSOCIATED WITH EXPLOSIVE BEHAVIOR

It is the premise of this book that explosive kids have lagging skills in the global domains of flexibility/adaptability, frustration tolerance, and problem solving. Developmental psychologists have long underscored the importance of these skills as related to a child's capacity to adapt to environmental changes or demands and to internalize standards of conduct (e.g., Crockenberg & Litman, 1990; Harter, 1983; Kochanska, 1993, 1995; Kopp, 1982, 1989; Rothbart & Derryberry, 1981). Capacities in these domains begin in infancy with managing the discomfort that can accompany hunger, cold, fatigue, and pain; modulating arousal while remaining engaged with the environment; and communicating with caregivers to signal that assistance is needed (e.g., Gottman, 1986; Kopp, 1989). More sophisticated mechanisms for flexibility/adaptability, frustration tolerance, and problem solving develop as children learn to use language to label and communicate their thoughts and feelings, develop cognitive schemas related to cause and effect, and generate and internalize strategies aimed at facilitating advantageous interactions with the environment (e.g., Kopp, 1989; Mischel, 1983). It is at around this point in development where two important forces—a child's capacity for compliance and adults' expectations for compliance—are thought to intersect. Researchers have underscored the frustration and emotional arousal that often accompany externally imposed demands for compliance (e.g., Amsel, 1990; Hoffman, 1975; Kochanska, 1993; Kopp, 1989; Stifter, Spinrad, & Braungart-Rieker, 1999). Indeed, the skill of compliance—

defined as the capacity to defer or delay one's own goals in response to the imposed goals or standards of an authority figure—can be considered one of many developmental expressions of the skills of flexibility/adaptability, frustration tolerance, and problem solving in young children (e.g., Maccoby, 1980; Perry & Perry, 1983; Stifter et al., 1999). Correspondingly, noncompliance can be understood as a byproduct of a developmental delay—a learning disability of sorts—in these domains, and helps explain why noncompliance and explosiveness so frequently coincide.

This conceptualization of noncompliance represents an important departure from conventional thinking and has equally important implications for treatment. In emphasizing *development* and *cognition*, the CPS model places a high priority on *identifying the specific cognitive factors contributing to the development of a given child's noncompliance and explosiveness*. Parents come into therapy asking, "What should I do with this child?" The CPS model proposes that this question cannot possibly be answered until a different question has been answered first: "What cognitive factors are contributing to this child's learning disability in the domains of flexibility/adaptability and frustration tolerance?"

The CPS model categorizes these cognitive factors into five clusters, or "pathways." We call these categories pathways because the lagging skills contained within each can set the stage for a child to head down the developmental "path" toward explosive behavior. Identifying the specific lagging skills underlying a child's explosive and noncompliant behavior accomplishes two crucial missions. First, adults are helped to understand that the child's difficulties are not due to a deficit in *motivation* or to *adult ineptitude* but rather to a deficit in *cognitive skills*, and therefore programs based on rewarding and punishing are unlikely to achieve satisfactory results because incentive-based programs do not train lacking cognitive skills. Second, adults are pointed directly to the specific cognitive skills that do need to be trained. Incidentally, diagnostic categories do not accomplish the latter mission satisfactorily because they lack descriptive specificity. For example, even if we are aware of the specific region of the brain that may have been affected, knowing that a child has a brain injury provides no information about the cognitive skills to be trained. Knowing that a child has ADHD, bipolar disorder, reactive attachment disorder, or any other disorder provides no information about the cognitive skills to be trained. Knowing that a child was born addicted to drugs or with fetal alcohol syndrome—while useful as a context for the child's present difficulties—provides no information about the cognitive skills to be trained now. Children with all of these conditions and diagnoses have lagging cognitive skills contained within the pathways, and the identification of these lagging skills is what truly pinpoints targets for intervention. Let's take a closer look at each pathway.

Executive Skills

While there is disagreement regarding the precise cognitive skills comprising the executive functions (see Lyon, 1996), there seems little disagreement regarding the detrimental effects of executive skill deficits on adaptive human functioning (see Douglas, 1980; Eslinger, 1996; Barkley, 1997a; Denckla, 1996; Fuster, 1995; Milner, 1995; Pennington & Ozonoff, 1996). A variety of cognitive skills have been characterized as "executive," including *working memory*, which refers to an individual's capacity to hold events in his or her mind while bringing to bear hindsight and forethought for the purpose of acting on the events (see Fuster, 1989, 1995; Pennington, 1994); *organization and planning*, which refer to an individual's capacity to organize his or her thoughts and inhibit impulses so as to define a problem, generate alternative solutions to the problem, and anticipate the likely outcomes of the solutions (see Borkowski & Burke, 1996); and *shifting cognitive set*, which refers to the efficiency and flexibility by which an individual shifts from the rules and expectations of one situation to the rules and expectations of another (see Hayes, Gifford, & Ruckstuhl, 1996).

Deficits in these domains have the potential to severely compromise a child's capacity to respond to adult directives in an adaptive (compliant) manner. Indeed, it has been shown that aggression rarely occurs outside the context of inattention and poor impulse control (e.g., Waschbusch, Willoughby, & Pelham, 1998), and this presumably explains the significant overlap between disorders associated with executive deficits (e.g., ADHD) and disorders associated with explosive behavior (i.e., ODD and CD) (Abikoff & Klein, 1992; Biederman, Faraone, Mick, et al., 1996; Hinshaw, Lahey, & Hart, 1993; Lahey & Loeber, 1994; Loeber & Keenan, 1994; Greene, Beszterczey, Katzenstein, Park, & Goring, 2002; Moffitt, 1990). For example, because adult directives typically require children to shift from the mind-set that immediately preceded the directive to the mind-set imposed by the adult, one might reasonably expect that a child compromised in the skill of shifting cognitive set would also be compromised in his or her capacity to comply rapidly with adult directives and might therefore experience greater than usual frustration were an adult to insist upon rapid compliance. A child challenged in working memory and/or planning might have difficulty efficiently reflecting upon both the previous consequences of noncompliance (hindsight) and the anticipated consequences of potential actions (forethought) in response to demands for rapid compliance, possibly contributing to the manifestation of any of a variety of behaviors that would be defined as explosive and noncompliant. Thus, explosive behavior may be better understood not as attention seeking, coercive, manipulative, or the by-product of lacking motivation, faulty learning, or inept parenting, but rather, at least partially, as the by-product of lagging cognitive skills.

Now, let us consider executive deficits in the context of a transactional conceptualization. It is clear that executive deficits do not guarantee that a child will evidence explosive behavior. From a transactional perspective, it is the degree of compatibility between a child with executive deficits and his adult caretakers that determines whether explosive (or other maladaptive) behaviors are ultimately expressed. If, for example, a child with executive deficits were "paired" with an adult who frequently imposed demands for rapid shifting of cognitive set and exhibited little tolerance for or understanding of slow or impulsive responding, we would predict a lower level of compatibility, at least in those interactions tapping into this combination of characteristics. By contrast, if the child were "paired" with an adult who was aware of this area of incompatibility, cognizant of the situations in which this incompatibility was likely to be most problematic, and interacted with the child in a way that mitigated this incompatibility, we would predict a higher level of compatibility.

Language-Processing Skills

As we have briefly discussed, language is crucial to the development of a variety of skills central to flexibility/adaptability and frustration tolerance (e.g., Bronowski, 1967, 1976, 1977; Luria, 1961; Piaget, 1952, 1981; Vygotsky, 1987). Not surprisingly, as many as half of all children who have language disorders also have psychiatric disorders (Cantwell & Baker, 1987, 1991), and there is a demonstrated association between language impairment and explosive behavior (Beitchman, Brownlie, & Wilson, 1996; Davis, Sanger, & Morris-Friehe, 1991; Gilmour, Hill, Place, & Skuse, 2004; Greene et al., 2002; Moffitt & Henry, 1991; Moffitt & Lynam, 1994).

Our experience is that lagging language-processing skills often go not only unnoticed but also unassessed. Yet skills such as labeling and categorizing one's emotions, communicating feelings and needs to others, sorting through and selecting response options, and receiving feedback about the appropriateness of one's actions are all crucial to dealing effectively with frustration and approaching problems in a flexible, adaptable manner—and are all mediated by language-processing skills (e.g., Bretherton, Fritz, Zahn-Waxler, & Ridgeway, 1986; Kopp, 1989). For example, children compromised in the capacity to label emotions may have difficulty developing and internalizing an adaptive repertoire of responses corresponding to emotions such as "sad" or "frustrated" or "disappointed." Children who lack the capacity to inform the world of their emotional state (e.g., "I'm frustrated") run the risk of being misinterpreted as "hostile," "scary," "out-of-control," or "aggressive," and may lack the linguistic wherewithal to correct the misinterpretations. Those who do not have the language skills to communicate about needs and problems can be expected to experience significant frustration in their attempts to get their needs met, alert others to problems, and participate in routine linguistic give-and-take. It can be persuasively argued that we humans rely almost exclusively on past experience to help us solve problems in the present, and that the problem-solving repertoires of children and adults are largely language based. Children with lagging language-processing skills may also evidence lags in accessing and contemplating potential solutions to problems and anticipating the likely outcomes and consequences of these solutions. Thus, as in the case of executive skills, explosive behavior may be better understood not as attention seeking, coercive, manipulative, or the by-product of lacking motivation or inept parenting but rather, at least partially, as the by-product of lacking cognitive skills . . . in this case, those related to language processing.

While language impairment heightens a child's risk for explosive behavior, such an outcome is by no means guaranteed. From a transactional perspective, once again, it is the degree of compatibility between a child with linguistic delays and his or her adult caretakers that determines whether explosive (or other maladaptive) behaviors are ultimately expressed. If a linguistically impaired child were, for example, paired with an adult who, while possibly aware of the child's language-processing difficulties, did not understand how these difficulties impacted the child's capacity for responding to simple requests, we would predict a lower level of compatibility, at least in those interactions tapping into this domain of their interactions. By contrast, if the child were matched with an adult who was aware of this area of incompatibility, cognizant of the situations in which this incompatibility was likely to be most problematic, and interacted with the child in a way that mitigated this incompatibility, we would predict a higher level of compatibility.

Emotion Regulation Skills

This category refers to a child's skills in regulating his acute emotional response to a given precipitant, as well as to a child's general or pervasive affective state.

As regards the former, the skill most frequently involved has been referred to as *separation of affect*, which is defined as an individual's capacity to regulate arousal in the service of goal-directed activity (Barkley, 1997a). Affect, of course, can be advantageous in that it serves the important function of energizing or mobilizing people to solve a problem, with thinking being the mechanism by which the problem is actually solved. However, too much affect can be an impediment to thinking and effective problem-solving. In practical terms, a child limited in the capacity to separate affect might respond to problems, frustrations, and anxieties with a high level of emotion (e.g., screaming, crying, swearing), thereby severely reducing his capacity for reasoned, reflective thinking. Indeed, many children find the emotional arousal associated with frustration difficult to modulate and tolerate and may therefore become cognitively debilitated in the midst of such arousal (a phenomenon referred to as "cognitive incapacitation" by Zillman, 1988). Various labels have been assigned to this arousal—often pegged to certain diagnoses—including the "affective storms" (prolonged and severe temper outbursts) seen in children said to have bipolar disorder (Wozniak & Biederman, 1996), and the "rage attacks" (explosive anger, irritability, temper outbursts, and aggression) described in children with Tourette's disorder (Budman, Bruun, Park, & Olson, 1998).

As regards a child's more general emotional state, here we are referring to a fairly chronic level of irritability, depression, and/or anxiety, for it is these affective states that can set the stage for the child to respond to minor routine frustrations—including demands for compliance—as if they were major obstacles, and therefore impede the acquisition of developmentally appropriate skills in the domains of flexibility/adaptability, frustration tolerance, and problem solving. This presumably explains the very high overlap between explosive behavior and disorders of mood (e.g., depression, bipolar disorder) and anxiety (Angold & Costello, 1993; Biederman, Faraone, Mick, et al., 1996; Bird, Gould, & Staghezza, 1993; Garland & Weiss, 1996; Geller & Luby, 1997; Greene et al., 2002; Harrington, Fudge, Rutter, Pickles, & Hill, 1991; Loeber & Keenan, 1994; Wozniak & Biederman, 1996; Zoccolillo, 1992).

In some circles, irritability, depression, and anxiety are thought to be purely driven by biology, thereby inspiring immediate consideration of pharmacological intervention. While pharmacotherapy can be an important component of treatment in youth in whom this pathway is implicated, it is important to underscore that such symptoms may have more to do with problematic life circumstances, or what we might think of as chronic problems that have never been solved. For example, a child's anxiety or irritability may be especially acute at school, because he is constantly teased or bullied or because of persistent (and perhaps unrecognized) learning inefficiencies. In such instances, helping the child solve the problems of teasing, bullying, or learning inefficiencies would conceivably make more sense than pharmacotherapy.

The important point, once again, is that explosive behavior may be better understood not as attention seeking, coercive, manipulative, or the by-product of lacking motivation or inept parenting, but rather, at least partially, as the by-product of lacking cognitive skills . . . in this case, those related to the regulation of emotions. How do such findings fit into a transactional conceptualization? As with executive and language-processing deficits, it is clear that emotion regulation difficulties do not guarantee that a child will develop explosive behavior. As we have mentioned before, it is the degree of compatibility between an irritable or anxious child and characteristics of his adult caretakers that determines whether explosive (or other maladaptive) behaviors are ultimately expressed. If an irritable or anxious child were paired with an adult who responded to the child in an impatient, inflexible, rigid manner, or misinterpreted the child's irritability as a "bad attitude," we might predict a low level of compatibility, at least as regards those interactions tapping into this combination of characteristics. By contrast, if the child were paired with an adult who was knowledgeable about and sensitive to the adult and child characteristics contributing to such incompatibility, aware of the situations in which this incompatibility was likely to be most problematic, and able to set the stage for interacting with the child in a way that mitigated this incompatibility, we would predict a higher level of compatibility.

Cognitive Flexibility Skills

Some children are extremely concrete, literal, black-and-white thinkers. Such kids tend to have very rigid templates for specific situations, can be very rule-oriented, often fail to take into account situational factors, and often focus on details rather than the "big picture." As one might expect, children with this profile tend to have strong preferences for predictability, routines, and rigid categorizations, and may experience significant frustration in circumstances of unpredictability and novelty or when events move outside of the norm or the expected. In practical terms, this is the child who may insist on going out for recess at a certain time on a given day because it is the time the class "always goes out for recess," failing to take into account both the likely outcome of insisting on the routine (e.g., being at recess alone) and important factors that would suggest the need for an adaptation in plan (e.g., a fire drill or an assembly). Such children may perseverate on or obsess over an idea or plan, and standard logic or reasoning frequently does not help the child shift gears. Social impairment is also common in such children; their literal approach to the world can make it difficult for them to appreciate subtle social cues and nuances, understand emotions in others, and appreciate the need for social reciprocity.

Black-and-white thinking may also adversely affect the manner by which a child interprets social information. Rigid, inaccurate, biased interpretations—sometimes referred to as cognitive distortions (Kendall, 1993)—may include beliefs such as "I'm stupid," "It's not fair," "You always blame me," "People are out to get me," "You can't trust adults," and "Nobody likes me." These beliefs—and the frustration that may accompany them—can heighten a child's level of arousal, narrow the accessibility and selection of response options (Akhtar & Bradley, 1991; Dodge, 1980, 1993; Dodge & Coie, 1987; Dodge, Price, Bachorowski, & Newman, 1990), and set the stage for any variety of maladaptive responses, including explosive outbursts.

A meaningful percentage of such children are diagnosed with nonverbal learning disability (NLD) or autism spectrum disorders (see Little, 1993; Rourke, 1989; Rourke & Fuerst, 1995; Semrud-Clikeman & Hynd, 1990), and data suggest that approximately 65% of children with autism spectrum disorders are also explosive and noncompliant (Greene et al., 2002). However, there are many concrete, literal, black-and-white children who do not satisfy criteria for a specific disorder. Regardless of diagnostic status, it should be clear that this profile can set the stage for significant difficulties in dealing adaptively with frustration and handling problems in a flexible, adaptable fashion.

As with the pathways reviewed above, explosive behavior in these kids may be better understood not as attention seeking, coercive, manipulative, or the by-product of lacking motivation or inept parenting but rather, at least partially, as the by-product of lacking cognitive skills . . . in this case, concrete, black-and-white, literal thinking. However, it is clear that while this profile heightens a child's risk for explosive behavior, yet again such an outcome is by no means guaranteed. Rather, we would predict heightened explosiveness if there were a lower degree of compatibility between the characteristics of these children and the characteristics of a given caregiver or social environment. A lower level of compatibility might be predicted, for example, if a literal thinker were paired with an adult who had a strong inclination toward sarcastic or highly nuanced communication. (We are reminded of the very literal child who became very agitated the first few times the therapist kindly asked him to come into the office and "take a seat"). By contrast, if the child were "paired" with an adult who was aware of this area of incompatibility, cognizant of the situations in which this incompatibility was likely to be most problematic, and interacted with the child in a way that mitigated this incompatibility, we would predict a higher level of compatibility.

Social Skills

Researchers have documented a significant overlap between social impairment and disruptive behavior disorders (e.g., Bloomquist, August, Cohen, Doyle, & Everhart, 1997; Dodge, 1993; Greene, Biederman, Faraone, Sienna, & Garcia-Jetton, 1997; Milich & Dodge, 1984; Moore, Hughes, & Robinson, 1992; Quiggle, Garber, Panak, & Dodge, 1992). Without commenting on the directionality of this overlap, it is not hard to understand how individuals compromised in the skills required for adaptive social interactions might also lag in the domains of flexibility/adaptability, frustration tolerance, and problem solving.

For example, researchers have shown that aggressive children are likely to have difficulties in social problem solving (e.g., Dodge, Pettit, McClaskey, & Brown, 1986; Lochman, White, & Wayland, 1991). Crucial skills often found lagging in socially impaired youth include recognizing the impact of one's behavior on others, comprehending how one is coming across, attending to social cues, and appreciating social nuances (Greene et al., 1997). Lagging skills in these important domains can impair a child's ability to gauge the appropriateness of their social behaviors and to accurately interpret, benefit from, and respond adaptively to social feedback. Those children impaired in pragmatic social skills may have difficulty sharing, entering a group, starting a conversation, taking turns in conversations, recognizing boredom in an interaction partner, regulating pitch and volume, and maintaining eye contact with and orientation to the speaker. It is not difficult to imagine how lagging skills in these domains may fuel, and limit a child's repertoire in dealing with, frustration, nor difficult to imagine how this frustration might be expressed.

Yet, as with the other pathways reviewed above, it is clear that while social impairment heightens a child's risk for explosive behavior, such an outcome is by no means guaranteed. Rather, we would predict higher levels of explosive (or other maladaptive) behaviors if there were a lower degree of compatibility between the socially impaired child and a given caregiver or social environment. A lower level of compatibility would be predicted if a child with a limited repertoire of social responses was paired with, for example, an adult who was overanxious about how the child was being perceived by others and overreactive about the child's poor social standing. By contrast, if the child was "paired" with an adult who was aware of this area of incompatibility, cognizant of the situations in which this incompatibility was likely to be most problematic, and interacted with the child in a way that mitigated this incompatibility, we would predict a higher level of compatibility.

The skills described above are enumerated in the Pathways Inventory

(Figure 1.1), a form we use as a framework for guiding questions in an initial clinical interview with adult caretakers. We discuss the Pathways Inventory in greater detail in Chapter 2. For now, it is worth reiterating that a major goal for clinicians implementing the CPS model is the assessment and identification of lagging thinking skills contributing to each child's difficulties for the purposes of helping caretakers understand that a child's explosions are neither purposeful nor intentional and helping pinpoint skills that will need to be trained.

ADULT CHARACTERISTICS ASSOCIATED WITH EXPLOSIVE BEHAVIOR

Let us now consider adult characteristics more fully. The difficulty in doing so, of course, is that the majority of research examining adult characteristics flows from unidirectional theories emphasizing inept parenting practices as the primary factor influencing the development of explosive behavior in children. In other words, a clear assumption about causality (parents are the primary agents influencing parent–child interactions) was the driving force in such research.

For example, Baumrind (e.g., 1968) found that *socially competent children* tend to have "authoritative" mothers (mothers who set a positive emotional context for parent–child interactions, characterized by warmth and nurturance, while still placing limits, demands, and controls). By contrast, *aggressive children* were found to have "permissive" mothers who responded to their children in an inconsistent manner, often failing to impose clear limits, especially when their children exhibited extreme negative behaviors or prolonged attempts to control them. *Anxious children* tended to have "authoritarian" mothers who were negative and punitive and showed little warmth and responsiveness but rather placed strict limits and controls that inhibited the development of their children's autonomy and social skills. These parenting styles differ on a power or control dimension, with authoritative mothers described as appropriately controlling, permissive mothers as undercontrolling, and authoritarian mothers as overcontrolling. If we were to be deeply invested in unidirectional explanations (which, of course, we are not), an alternative unidirectional interpretation of these adult characteristics is possible: socially competent children elicit far greater warmth and nurturance from their parents than children who are less socially competent. Fortunately, by emphasizing cognition, development, and compatibility, such "chicken versus egg" debates lose their appeal.

In our experience, parents of explosive children are as varied as their children. Indeed, we find that many of the characteristics of children that contribute to explosive adult–child interchanges are found in their parents as well. We find executive difficulties and problems with emotion regulation in many of the adults with whom we work; we also find language-processing issues, black-and-white thinking, and cognitive deficiencies and distortions. As by-products of these characteristics, we find that many adults have difficulty prioritizing and deciding about the relative importance of their parenting goals. We find that other adults bring very rigid definitions regarding adult "authority" to parent–child interactions, leaving no option for discussion, processing, "meeting halfway," or inviting the child to participate jointly in solving problems. Other adults have a limited or rigid repertoire of options for pursuing the behavioral goals they have set for their children. Still other adults have difficulty envisioning and anticipating the likely outcomes of their options. Some adults have abandoned most of their parenting agenda, often so as to avoid an overreactive, aversive response from their child. Others run a household and parent in a manner that is disorganized, unstructured, and haphazard, leading to impulsive parenting decisions. Yet others are highly irritable, have little energy to devote to what some would consider routine issues of parenting, and often overreact to child behaviors that might not fall outside of what would be considered developmentally appropriate. If we are to improve adult–child incompatibility, it will certainly be necessary to incorporate these adult characteristics into our treatment plans (without making assumptions about causality).

*   *   *

In its emphasis on assessing, identifying, and remediating lagging cognitive skills, the CPS model is grounded in social learning theory. Yet in many respects, the model represents a fairly significant departure from conventional wisdom in conceptualizing and treating kids with behavioral challenges. In Chapter 2 we focus on the pragmatics of assessing and identifying lagging cognitive skills contributing to adult–child conflict. In Chapters 3–6 we describe the CPS model of intervention in greater detail, especially as it would be implemented in an outpatient setting. In the subsequent two chapters, we focus on implementation of CPS in general education schools (Chapter 7) and therapeutic/restrictive facilities (Chapter 8). The information presented in Chapters 2–6 is highly relevant to individuals working in these settings. Indeed, the content presented in Chapters 7 and 8 will make little sense unless the preceding chapters have been read first. Finally, in Chapter 9 we provide answers to a lot of the questions clinicians and researchers have about the model and describe early studies examining the efficacy of the CPS approach.

Executive skills
____ Difficulty handling transitions, shifting from one mindset or task to another, adapting to new circumstances or rules
____ Poor sense of time/difficulty doing things in a logical or prescribed order
____ Disorganized/difficulty staying on topic, sorting through thoughts, or keeping track of things
____ Difficulty considering the likely outcomes or consequences of actions (impulsive)
____ Difficulty considering a range of solutions to a problem

Language-processing skills
____ Often has difficulty expressing thoughts, needs, or concerns in words
____ Often appears not to have understood what was said
____ Long delays before responding to questions
____ Difficulty knowing or saying how he/she feels

Emotion regulation skills
____ Difficulty staying calm enough to think rationally (when frustrated)
____ Cranky, grouchy, grumpy, irritable (outside the context of frustration)
____ Sad, fatigued, tired, low energy
____ Anxious, nervous, worried, fearful

Cognitive flexibility skills
____ Concrete, black-and-white, thinker; often takes things literally
____ Insistence on sticking with rules, routine, original plan
____ Does poorly in circumstances of unpredictability, ambiguity, uncertainty
____ Difficulty shifting from original idea or solution; possibly perseverative or obsessive
____ Difficulty appreciating another person's perspective or point-of-view
____ Doesn't take into account situational factors that would suggest the need to adjust a plan of action
____ Inflexible, inaccurate interpretations/cognitive distortions or biases (e.g., "Everyone's out to get me," "Nobody likes me," "You always blame me," "It's not fair," "I'm stupid," "Things will never work out for me")

Social skills
____ Difficulty attending to or misreading of social cues/poor perception of social nuances/difficulty recognizing nonverbal social cues
____ Lacks basic social skills (how to start a conversation, how to enter a group, how to connect with people)
____ Seeks the attention of others in inappropriate ways; seems to lack the skills to seek attention in an adaptive fashion
____ Seems *unaware* of how behavior is affecting other people; is surprised by others' responses to his/her behavior
____ Lacks empathy; appears *not to care* about how behavior is affecting others or their reactions
____ Poor sense of how s/he is coming across or being perceived by others
____ Inaccurate self-perception

Triggers (list)
1.
2.
3.

FIGURE 1.1. Pathways Inventory.

Chapter 2

Identifying Pathways and Triggers

In Chapter 1, we delineated several important core principles of the CPS model. Foremost among these principles is the notion that explosive behavior is the by-product of incompatibility between characteristics of children and their adult caretakers. Also paramount is the notion that child and adult characteristics are best understood and captured in the context of their respective cognitive skills. We delineated five domains (pathways) that we find useful for categorizing these cognitive skills, including executive skills, emotion regulation skills, language-processing skills, cognitive flexibility skills, and social skills. Embedded within each pathway are specific cognitive skills that may be lacking (i.e., "skills that need to be trained"). As we've described, a crucial first goal of intervention is to assess and identify the skill deficits that best explain a given child's explosive behavior (and the behavior of his adult caretakers). A simultaneous goal is the identification of *triggers* that commonly precipitate explosive episodes (e.g., sensory hypersensitivities, homework, sharing, reading, writing, getting ready for school in the morning, getting ready for bed at night, interacting with a particular classmate or sibling). Triggers are best conceived as "problems that have yet to be solved."

Once pathways and triggers have been identified, explosive episodes become highly predictable. This is a crucial point of emphasis, for the CPS model places almost exclusive emphasis on *antecedent events* (what adults do proactively to prevent explosive episodes) rather than on consequences (what adults do reactively, or after the fact, to manage such episodes). Although this is not a radical concept theoretically (behaviorists have always emphasized the importance of focusing on antecedents), in practice we find that a concentration on antecedents represents a major shift for many clinicians. If explosive episodes are predictable, then the stage is set for proactive discussion and resolution of the problems that cause such episodes. By the way, a trigger does not have to set the stage for an explosive episode with 100% reliability to be of interest. A trigger simply needs to *heighten the likelihood* of such an episode to be of interest.

SITUATIONAL ANALYSIS

In general, there are two mechanisms by which pathways and triggers can be identified: a clinical interview and, in some cases, a more formal assessment. As regards the latter, we tend to rely on pediatric neuropsychologists to accomplish the mission. The information provided by formal testing can often be helpful in clarifying cognitive skills and inefficiencies, especially in the domains of executive skills, language-processing skills, cognitive flexibility skills, and memory. Data provided by such assessments can also provide useful information about a child's general cognitive skills and potential triggers (e.g., skill deficits in specific academic domains, such as reading, spelling, mathematics, and written language).

As regards the former, we employ two tools. The first—the Pathways Inventory—was introduced in Chapter 1, and is a very useful instrument for guiding interviews with caretakers aimed at identifying the lagging cognitive skills that may be contributing to explosive episodes. The word "interview" is important here, for we find the Pathways Inventory to be far less useful when it is used as a checklist (items that are endorsed in checklist format need to be fleshed out and clarified in ways that checklists do not permit). We also find that those new to the Pathways Inventory tend to treat the five pathway categories as diagnoses and tend to prioritize those categories with the most items endorsed. We discourage this use of the Pathways Inventory as well, as we find that global categorizations do not afford a sufficient level of specificity. Only identifying specific lagging skills provides the necessary level of specificity. Moreover, counting items under each category isn't a terribly useful way to prioritize; determining which specific skills are contributing to the most explosive episodes tends to be far more productive.

The second tool—the situational analysis—is also useful for identifying pathways and triggers. Explosive episodes occur only under certain circumstances (Hoffenaar, 2004). More specifically, such outbursts occur exclusively in situations of heightened levels of incompatibility between a child and the environment (in other words, when a demand is placed upon a child that exceeds the child's capacity to respond adaptively). Thus, identifying these situations is absolutely essential, and requires an early focus on the question *"In what situations do explosive episodes occur, and what do these situations tell us about cognitive factors and triggers contributing to incompatibility and non-compliance?"* In pursuing this question, be forewarned: since most adults do not think about children's maladaptive behavior in situational terms, be prepared for some detective work. Nonetheless, situations in which explosive episodes occur provide rich information about the triggers that may routinely and predictably precipitate such episodes and about the cognitive characteristics of the interaction partners who were involved.

When we first meet with a child's adult caretakers, we commonly ask for a description of the child's explosive episodes. While we are not primarily interested in what a child *does* during such episodes, we know it is important to many adults to have the opportunity to describe the unsettling and sometimes scary behaviors a child may evidence (e.g., hitting, kicking, spitting, throwing, swearing, screaming, etc.), and we also like to get a sense of the degree to which a child's behavior may be considered unsafe. We find that adults often don't need large doses of empathy in response to such descriptions; they mostly need to be *believed*. Indeed, we think the best way to demonstrate empathy is by asking questions that communicate an understanding of explosive children and an ability to home in on the factors underlying a given child's explosive episodes. Once again, what we are looking for is information that will help us identify the pathways and triggers underlying explosive episodes.

Toward this end, we typically ask caretakers to describe several recent explosive episodes, with the primary goal of making sense out of each story in terms of the lagging skills and triggers that might best account for what transpired. Our motto: *A story is just a story unless you use it to identify a pathway or a trigger.* In other words, contained within each story is information about cognitive skills that a child (or his adult caretakers) lacks or precipitants that heighten his (or their) frustration. And although many of the details of a story might be interesting, the most important details are those that help clarify the pathways or triggers. Thus, when we listen to stories, we ask reporters, "Does this situation commonly cause explosive episodes?" And we commonly ask ourselves, "What cognitive skill would have been required for handling that situation adaptively?" We feel reasonably safe in hypothesizing that a child's difficulties are being fueled by a particular pathway if that pathway is implicated in many explosive episodes.

In an initial meeting in outpatient therapy, we typically meet first with caretakers (without the child in the room), then with the child (without the caretakers in the room), and then try to assess family dynamics with the caretakers and child in the room together. Here's how the combination of a situational analysis and use of the Pathways Inventory might sound in an initial meeting with a parent (in reading the foregoing dialogue, you might wish to reflect on the pathways described in Chapter 1 so as to come to your own hypotheses about the pathways and triggers that are coming into play). Note that this dialogue is not as detailed as would normally be the case, but it does provide a good example of the general line of inquiry:

THERAPIST: Tell me about Janet's explosions.

PARENT: Oh my, what do you want to know?

THERAPIST: I think it would be useful to get specific about when Janet explodes . . . you know, who she's with, what she's having difficulty with, and so forth.

PARENT: I don't understand what you mean.

THERAPIST: Well, from what I can gather, Janet isn't having explosive episodes every second of every waking hour. She's explosive and noncompliant sometimes . . . with some people, on some tasks, during some times of the day. If we can figure out when those "sometimes" are, we'll have a much better chance of understanding what's causing the episodes and then we can begin working on keeping them from happening.

PARENT: I don't think there ever is a reason . . . she just goes nuts.

THERAPIST: We sometimes hear that a child explodes for no apparent reason. But, I must say, our experience is that outbursts don't usually happen in a "vacuum" . . . there's usually a reason, usually something that sets the child off. So maybe you could tell me about some recent blowups.

PARENT: Hmm . . . well, yesterday she went completely nuts because her younger brother was annoying her in the car. Is that what you mean?

THERAPIST: I think so. Do you think it was the car ride or was it her brother annoying her that set her off?

PARENT: You lost me again.

THERAPIST: I'm just wondering which was more problematic for Janet . . . riding in the car or her brother annoying her?

PARENT: Oh, I gotcha. No, she doesn't mind riding in the car. But she finds her brother to be very annoying.

THERAPIST: Did Janet say anything about what her brother was doing that was so annoying?

PARENT: I guess he was just being a little hyper.

THERAPIST: Was he making lots of noise, was he moving around a lot . . . ?

PARENT: I think he was bumping up against her.

THERAPIST: OK, so her brother is bumping up against her in the car . . . how did Janet respond to that?

PARENT: She just started screaming that she wanted him to stop bumping up against her. Is that helpful?

THERAPIST: Possibly. Is she often easily annoyed by little things like that?

PARENT: Like what? Her brother bumping up against her?

THERAPIST: I guess what I'm trying to get a handle on is whether Janet is easily annoyed a lot of the time or whether there was something particularly annoying about being bumped by her brother.

Having ruled out car rides as a trigger, the therapist is trying to home in on whether this explosive episode is most easily understood with a pathway (emotion regulation) or a trigger (either sensory issues or interactions with the brother).

PARENT: Well, she's never very patient with her brother . . . but she's a pretty grumpy kid to begin with.

THERAPIST: Are there other times she's grumpy besides when she's with her brother?

PARENT: I guess I've always thought she was pretty grumpy all the time— although her teachers think she's an absolute delight.

THERAPIST: So she's mostly grumpy at home?

PARENT: Yes—you know, we didn't know how grumpy she really was until we had my son. He's about as happy and easygoing as they come.

THERAPIST: Would you say she's grumpy only when she's frustrated, or is she grumpy even when she's not frustrated?

PARENT: That's an interesting question . . . I'd say she's grumpy even when she's not frustrated. She's a bear when she wakes up in the morning.

THERAPIST: Any other times of the day that you've noticed she's especially grumpy or irritable?

PARENT: She's deadly when she gets home from school. It's almost like she's put so much energy into holding it together at school that she's got nothing left when she gets home.

THERAPIST: That's something we see a lot. How can you tell she's grumpy when she gets home from school?

PARENT: She's surly . . . and very disagreeable . . . it's easiest just to leave her alone for a while.

We're getting a strong signal for irritability (emotion regulation pathway), although we would want greater clarification on why the irritability predominantly occurs at home. Let's explore the emotion regulation pathway a bit further and then move on to other pathways and triggers.

THERAPIST: Well, I'm getting the strong sense that she's grumpy and irritable a lot. Would you agree?

PARENT: Absolutely. Does that mean she has bipolar disorder?

THERAPIST: What makes you think she has bipolar disorder?

PARENT: I was reading some things on the Internet.

THERAPIST: Well, we can talk about diagnoses as I get to know her a little better, but right now I'm just trying to get a sense for why she's so inflexible and responds to frustration so poorly.

(Just because a parent thinks a diagnosis will be useful doesn't mean he or she is right! Even when a child meets criteria for a diagnosis, our focus on triggers and lagging skills is unaltered.)

THERAPIST: Do you find that she's nervous or worried a lot?

PARENT: Well . . . she gets a little nervous before tests . . . but nothing off the charts. No, I guess I don't think of her as being particularly nervous or worried a lot.

THERAPIST: OK, let's go back to the car for a moment . . . aside from being grumpy and easily annoyed, is there anything else about being bumped by her brother that might have set her off?

PARENT: Like what?

THERAPIST: I guess I was wondering if maybe she's oversensitive to people making physical contact with her in general, or whether there are other physical stimuli that bother her.

PARENT: Other physical stimuli?

THERAPIST: Things like the feel of clothing, tags in clothing, bright lights, loud noises . . . ?

PARENT: Well, now, she's always been bothered by people touching her . . . she likes hugs, but they have to be on her terms . . . I mean, she has to be "ready" for them. And she hates feeling "crowded. " You should have seen how hot and bothered she was standing in lines at Disney World. That was not fun.

THERAPIST: I can imagine. But clothing and lights and noises . . . nothing big there?

PARENT: You know, now that I think of it, she has always been very particular about the clothes she's willing to wear . . . she hates things that are tight or itchy . . . seams in her socks used to drive her crazy. I guess I never gave it a lot of thought.

Sensory hypersensitivities appear to be an important trigger. Let's plunge forward.

THERAPIST: Can you tell me about anything else she's blown up over in the past few weeks?

PARENT: But what am I supposed to do when she gets upset in the car? I mean, she's tough to deal with in the first place, but having her lose it while I'm on the highway is dangerous!

THERAPIST: I agree. I think you'll have some ideas on how to handle that before you leave today, but for now I want to see if I can get the best possible sense of the types of things that set her off. Until I know what's causing the difficulties, I won't know how to help you fix the problem.

Note that the therapist doesn't feel she can offer any credible guidance on intervention until she has a better sense of what she's dealing with.

THERAPIST: Got any more stories?

PARENT: Well, homework is a daily disaster.

THERAPIST: Tell me what goes on during homework.

PARENT: She's always saying it's too noisy in the house for her to get her work done.

THERAPIST: Too noisy? Is she right?

PARENT: (*laughing*) She does her homework in a quiet part of the house, and she'll go nuts if she hears me and her brother *whispering* at the other end of the house! She says it messes up her concentration! I can't take her brother out of the house for 4 hours every afternoon while she does her homework!

THERAPIST: No, that doesn't sound like a very realistic solution to that problem. Just to make sure I understand, what Janet says is making her upset is noises, yes?

PARENT: *Any* noises!

THERAPIST: So the issue isn't that Janet doesn't want to do her homework, it's that she feels like she's being disturbed while she's trying to do it, yes?

PARENT: Oh, she wants to do her homework . . . she's a very hard worker in school . . . I will say homework takes her much longer than her teachers say it's supposed to.

THERAPIST: How long is she supposed to do homework every night?

PARENT: According to her teachers, about 90 minutes.

THERAPIST: 90 minutes? And it's taking her 4 hours?

PARENT: Yup.

THERAPIST: What do we make of that?

PARENT: I was hoping you'd make something out of it.

THERAPIST: I suppose there are lots of possibilities. Is it too hard for her?

PARENT: I doubt it. This kid is *very* smart.

THERAPIST: I get a lot of kids through here who are very smart but who still have learning issues that are slowing them down in specific ways that have nothing to do with their intelligence.

PARENT: She's had testing . . . and the school said she's at least average in everything and almost a genius in a lot of areas.

THERAPIST: Hmm. Still, it's taking her 4 hours to do homework that is only supposed to take 90 minutes. Why don't I take a look at the test reports you brought with you. . . . Well, the first thing I'm noticing here is that Janet has exceptional verbal skills—this 132 score tells me that. But her nonverbal skills are not as well developed—this 98 score tells me that.

PARENT: The school said not to worry about the 98 because it was still average.

THERAPIST: Well, they were right in saying it was average, but that doesn't necessarily mean it's nothing to worry about. That 34-point discrepancy—between her verbal skills and her nonverbal skills—may tell us something about why Janet is taking so long to get her homework done and why she gets so frustrated. Tell me, would you describe her as a very rigid kid?

PARENT: I don't know what you mean.

THERAPIST: Is she a very concrete, black-and-white, literal thinker? Does she insist that things always be a certain way? Does she get an idea in her head and it would take an earthquake to shake it loose?

PARENT: You mean the type of kid who insists that others follow certain rules?

THERAPIST: Something like that . . . a kid who has certain pretty rigid ideas about the way things are supposed to be and wants everyone else to stick to those ideas.

PARENT: Oh, God, you just hit the nail on the head. One of the reasons she has trouble keeping friends is that she's always correcting them when they do something wrong or bossing them around when they don't do things the way she wants them to. And around the house, she's got rules for how family members should behave and goes nuts when we don't follow her rules.

THERAPIST: I wonder if homework is taking a long time because Janet is very rigid about the way it's supposed to be done. She might also have very rigid ideas about how quiet things are supposed to be during homework. What do you think?

PARENT: I don't know . . . I mean, I've never thought about it that way. I just figured she's easily bothered by noises.

THERAPIST: That could be part of it, too . . . but her testing profile and what little I've heard about how she interacts with other kids suggest there may be more to it than that. She may be able to provide some information about this when I meet with her.

PARENT: I thought I was just dealing with "superbrat."

THERAPIST: Well, I guess the key point here is that while she probably comes across as "superbrat," there are some real issues related to how she thinks that are making it very difficult for her to interact with the world. Tell me, what else makes you think she's very rigid and black and white?

PARENT: I'll tell you a story. The other day I'm driving her home from soccer practice. I'm thinking it might be nice to take a different way home. She goes ballistic because we're not going the way we usually go. I'm thinking, "I can't believe I'm living with someone who goes ballistic when we don't go the exact way we usually go."

THERAPIST: OK, I'm sold. And you're right, that's extremely difficult to live with. Of course, it probably makes life extremely difficult for Janet as well.

PARENT: Oh, I'm sure. I feel bad for her. I mean, I know she's not doing this stuff on purpose, but it's hard to remember that when you're in the middle of her going ballistic.

Rigid, black-and-white thinking (cognitive flexibility pathway) appears to be a major contributor to Janet's inflexibility, poor tolerance for frustration, and difficulties with problem solving. Let's explore the remaining pathways.

THERAPIST: You mentioned a few minutes ago that she has difficulty keeping friends because she's always correcting them. Can you give me a general sense of how things are going for her socially?

PARENT: Not terrible, but not great. You know, she really wants friends, and she tries very hard to make them. It's just that she's very critical, and very bossy.

THERAPIST: Does she have friends?

PARENT: Not as many as she thinks she does. But there is one girl she's been friends with since the first grade and they stay friends no matter how badly Janet treats her.

THERAPIST: Aside from being bossy and critical and always correcting people, are there other things that seem to be getting in the way for Janet socially?

PARENT: Like what?

THERAPIST: I'm wondering how she is at taking other people's perspective, being aware of how she's coming across . . .

PARENT: Not good. She loves animals . . . she can take a dog's perspective . . . but I don't think she's ever been very good at knowing how she makes other people feel or how she comes across.

THERAPIST: Are there any other things about how she interacts with people that causes her difficulty?

PARENT: How do you mean?

THERAPIST: Well, does she have a hard time reading social cues—like facial expressions, or people being bored with what she's saying—or does she have a hard time knowing how to join a group or keep a conversation going with a friend?

PARENT: No . . . not really. I mean, I think the main thing is that she just wants everything to be her way.

While there is action on the social skills pathway, the therapist has placed this pathway on the back burner, at least temporarily, because it doesn't seem to be a major factor as regards explosive episodes.

THERAPIST: OK, let me just ask about a few more things. Do people complain that Janet is overactive, or impulsive, or has trouble focusing in school?

PARENT: Oh, you mean ADHD? No, her teachers say she's very focused. And I've never thought of her as hyper.

THERAPIST: So you don't think a possible explanation for why she's taking so long with her homework is because she's having trouble staying focused?

PARENT: I always thought it was just the noise.

THERAPIST: Let me look at the testing again . . . they're not saying anything about her having trouble focusing . . . but I am seeing that her scores in arithmetic and written expression are in the mid-90s. Does her homework involve a lot of math or writing?

PARENT: Not so much math, but a ton of writing. The school told me her scores in math and writing were average.

THERAPIST: There's that word again. "Average" compared to other kids, maybe. "Average" compared to what her IQ tells us to expect from Janet, no.

PARENT: I've offered to help her with her writing assignments, but she just screams at me that I'll make things worse.

THERAPIST: Maybe there is some form of help that she might find to be more acceptable . . . we'll find out. In the meantime, I think we may end up having some discussions with the folks at school to find out what type of assistance they might be able to offer.

PARENT: But they don't even think she needs help.

THERAPIST: Yes, that will be an important area of discussion as well. But if it takes her more than twice as long as it should to finish her homework, that's probably a sign that something is wrong.

Another potential trigger—written language—has been identified. So we've now identified two primary pathway areas (irritability and concrete, black-and-white thinking) and two major triggers (sensory issues and home-work/written language).

THERAPIST: OK, let me ask you a few more questions. I'm seeing that the previous testing did not include a speech and language assessment. Am I missing something, or was it not done?

PARENT: I don't think she's ever had a speech and language assessment. Why, do you think she needs one?

THERAPIST: I don't know. Have you ever noticed that Janet has any difficulty saying what she wants to say or understanding what other people are saying?

PARENT: I've never really noticed . . . I don't think so . . . no, I'd say she's pretty good at saying what she wants to say. She has a great vocabulary. She's never given me the impression that she isn't understanding something I'm saying.

THERAPIST: OK . . . I'll assess that informally when I meet with her anyway and then I'll have a better idea about whether formal assessment is needed. But I think we have some pretty good clues about why Janet is so inflexible and handles frustration so poorly. I'm getting the very strong sense that Janet's irritability is more chronic and intense than would be expected for a child her age, and I know how inflexible and easily frustrated most people are when they're in an irritable, grumpy mood. Problem is, Janet's in an irritable, grumpy mood a lot and that may be setting the stage for her to be inflexible and easily frustrated a lot. Now what we don't know yet is the degree to which her difficulties with schoolwork are having a significant impact on her mood. That's something we'll have to assess as we go along. It's possible that her mood will improve if we solve some of the problems—homework, writ-ing, sensory sensitivities—that are causing her frustration.

PARENT: OK. How do we solve them?

THERAPIST: We're almost there. I'm also hearing that Janet is a very con-crete, black-and-white thinker . . . once she has an idea in her head it's extremely difficult to move her in a different direction. It also sounds like things are a bit difficult for her socially; as we see in many concrete, black-and-white thinking kids, she has a lot of trouble taking the perspective of other people and understanding how she's coming across, and those are things that often make it difficult to make and keep friends. It's not clear to me that her social issues are causing a lot of explosions, and I don't know how troubling it is to her that she has difficulties getting along with other kids.

PARENT: I'm not sure she even knows.

THERAPIST: Exactly. I'm not getting a strong signal on executive skills. Nor am I getting a strong signal on language, although that's one we'll want to gather at least a little more information on.

Having achieved an initial sense of the triggers precipitating Janet's explosive episodes and the lagging cognitive skills setting the stage for the episodes, and having provided Janet's mother with an initial impression along these lines, the therapist is about to ask a crucial question ("Does this sound like Janet to you?"). If the question is responded to in the affirmative, then the therapist has begun to accomplish two of the important missions described in Chapter 1: first, adults have been helped to understand that the child's difficulties are not due to a deficit in *motivation* but rather to a deficit in *skills*; second, adults have been helped to pinpoint the specific cognitive skills that need to be trained.

THERAPIST: Does this sound like Janet to you?

PARENT: Wow . . . I mean, yes. She has a lot going on, doesn't she?

THERAPIST: I'd say we've got our work cut out for us.

PARENT: But what does it all mean? Where do we start?

THERAPIST: Well, now that we have a bit of a sense about the factors contributing to Janet's outbursts, we also have a clearer sense about the things we need to work on so she doesn't have the outbursts anymore. Those factors also make it easier for us to predict explosions in advance.

PARENT: So we need to work on her irritability and black-and-white thinking?

THERAPIST: Right. And find solutions to the problems that haven't been solved yet . . . the ones that are jumping out at me right now are homework and sensory stimuli.

PARENT: How?

THERAPIST: We're getting there, I promise. But understanding why she has these outbursts is a huge step.

PARENT: And you're saying we can predict her explosions? I always thought they were so out of the blue.

THERAPIST: A lot of folks tell us the episodes seem like they're out of the blue, but that theory is usually proven false. Janet is actually beginning to sound like a very predictable kid.

The above "sound bite" illustrates how much can be accomplished through conducting a situational analysis and by sticking closely to the task of identifying lagging cognitive skills and triggers. Note that the therapist does-n't discuss the pathways in terms of *general categories* (e.g., executive skills, emotion regulation skills, etc.), but rather in terms of the *specific skills* contained within each pathway that appear to apply to the child. Naturally, other important information would be gathered in the initial interview with caretakers, such as the pharmacological and psychosocial treatment history of the child and other family members, marital issues, other family stressors, history of parental interactions with the child's school, and the manner by which adults have historically responded to problems or unmet expectations. As regards this latter line of inquiry, let's listen in once more.

THERAPIST: Tell me, how have you typically handled Janet when she becomes upset?

PARENT: You mean after everyone stops screaming? We tell her we're not going to tolerate disrespectful behavior and then she usually gets some sort of punishment. Then there's usually more screaming.

THERAPIST: I'm assuming you'd like to cut back on the screaming.

PARENT: That's why I'm here.

THERAPIST: The big question is whether telling Janet you're not going to tolerate disrespectful behavior and punishing her has been effective.

PARENT: Depends who you ask.

THERAPIST: How do you mean?

PARENT: Well, her father—he actually did want to be here today, but he had an emergency at work—he thinks she has to be taught that we're not going to tolerate her outbursts.

THERAPIST: If what he means by that is that we need to find some way to significantly reduce Janet's outbursts, then I'd agree with him. Problem is,

I don't think punishment is going to get the job done. What do you think?

PARENT: Well, I've always had the sense that something's the matter with Janet that we just hadn't figured out yet. And you seem to be saying the same thing.

THERAPIST: I'm saying that Janet has a great deal of difficulty dealing with frustration, being flexible, and solving problems, and, now that we've talked, I think we have a better sense of why that might be. The reason punishment hasn't worked is that it doesn't fix the things that are causing Janet to have difficulty in the first place. Punishment doesn't help her be less irritable, doesn't help her be less of a black-and-white thinker, doesn't address her sensory issues, and doesn't help her with her homework. If we solve those problems, you, your husband, and Janet will be fighting a lot less.

Of course, generating hypotheses about pathways and triggers can also be facilitated by an interview with the child. Such interviews differ dramatically based on the age and attitude of the child. All the usual early interviewing goals are still relevant: helping a child feel comfortable, laying the foundation for a therapeutic alliance, and so forth. Frequently, our first question to a child or adolescent is, "What did your parents tell you about why they were dragging you here today?" Although this question is frequently responded to with a shrug or "I don't know," the goal is to begin a brief discussion about the difficulties family members are having in getting along with each other. It is important to establish (directly or indirectly) that we do not view the child or adolescent as the "problem" or the "identified patient." The *family* is the identified patient. While there may be some discussion of problems the child is having with his or her "temper" or in handling frustration, it is extremely important for these discussions to remain blameless. In the case of adolescents who may be irritated at having been dragged to yet another therapist's office, we might go a bit overboard to form an alliance by asking, "Tell me what's the matter with your parents." Adolescents frequently find this line of inquiry to be a refreshing departure from their experiences with prior therapists.

THERAPIST: Why'd your parents drag you here today?

ADOLESCENT: 'Cause they're messed up.

THERAPIST: How are they messed up?

ADOLESCENT: Look, I really do not feel like doing this right now.

THERAPIST: I guess you've got better things to be doing right now than talk-ing to a stranger about the problems you're having with your parents.

ADOLESCENT: You guess right.

THERAPIST: Can I take another guess?

ADOLESCENT: Whatever floats your boat.

THERAPIST: I'm guessing you've done this many times before.

ADOLESCENT: Done what? Had them make me talk to some shrink?

THERAPIST: Yeah, that.

ADOLESCENT: Hell, yes. I've lost count. It's a waste of my freaking time. Never done me a bit of good.

THERAPIST: Well, then I can understand you thinking that this will be a com-plete waste of your time.

ADOLESCENT: Thank you very much.

THERAPIST: The way I figure it, if any of the doctors you'd seen before had done you guys any good, you all wouldn't be here right now.

ADOLESCENT: Exactly.

THERAPIST: So here's the deal. I don't know if I can do you guys any good or not. You've been fighting with each other for a very long time. That's not an easy thing to fix, and I'm not the type to make promises I can't keep. But I won't know if I can help unless you tell me what's the mat-ter with your parents and why you all keep fighting so much.

ADOLESCENT: 'Cause they're f——ed up.

THERAPIST: Give me some details. I don't know exactly what you mean.

ADOLESCENT: They're too f——ing strict, they don't know squat about kids, they're always on my case, they're always pissed off about some-thing . . . get the idea?

THERAPIST: I do. Sounds unpleasant. Can you fill me in on what they're so strict about?

Ultimately, we are seeking the child's independent report on the situa-tions that are causing conflict (triggers) and perhaps some information about the lagging skills contributing to such conflict. To assess triggers, we might ask, "What do you and your parents (or teachers) fight (or disagree) about the most?" or "Do you ever get really mad at your parents (or teachers)? About what?" To assess specific skills, we might ask: "Do you find that it's hard for you to pay attention in school?"; "Do you get into trouble a lot because it's hard for you to sit still or you're calling out in class?"; "Do you ever find that it's hard for you to understand what other people are saying or hard for you to put what you want to say into words?"; "What kind of mood are you in most of the time?"; "Would you describe yourself as very nervous or worried a lot of the time? About what?"; "Tell me about how things are going with friends. Do you have as many as you'd like? What seems to be getting in the way?"; "Do you get very upset if things don't go a certain way?" Naturally, the therapist's observations of a child's capacity for linguistic give-and-take, interest in connecting, general social skills, problem solving, self-regulation, and flexibility can be as important as a child's actual answers to these questions.

As noted earlier, in many instances, critical information about the pathways can also be provided by formal testing. Sometimes such testing has already been performed, and sometimes the prior testing is of adequate quality. But in some cases a referral to a competent pediatric neuropsychologist, speech and language pathologist, and/or occupational therapist is indicated. There are excellent resources providing highly detailed descriptions of the goals of such assessment and the instrumentation used to achieve these goals (e.g., Culbertson & Willis, 1992), so such details are not provided here.

Let's return to an important point. In the preceding dialogue with Janet's mother we noted that we find it useful to summarize our hypotheses about a child's lacking skills and the manner by which they are contributing to a child's difficulties in the domains of flexibility/adaptability, frustration tolerance, and problem solving. This summary is provided to the adults in terms aimed at describing a child's cognitive deficits rather than at diagnosing the child. For a few reasons, we always present our early impressions as just that: *early impressions* or *working hypotheses*. First, initial clinical impressions are based on incomplete information. Second, pretending that we can, in just one hour, come to highly definitive conclusions about the factors underlying a child's difficulties sends the wrong message. Indeed, we think clinicians demonstrate expertise far more effectively by being honest about the difficulties inherent in comprehensively understanding a child than by being falsely (and therefore often erroneously) definitive.

It goes without saying that assessment—coming to a more definitive understanding of triggers and pathways—is a continuous and ongoing process of treatment. However, as depicted above, after presenting our hypotheses to the adults, we ask whether our impressions make sense to them and whether they are consistent with their own observations and understanding of their child. Again, once adults have "signed on" to our early impressions of a given child, a few important things happen. First, we now have a *consensus*. Discussions and decisions about intervention options can now proceed in an educated fashion with some common assumptions about the factors underlying a child's difficulties. All too often, discussions and decisions about intervention march forward before caretakers have come to a consensus about the nature of a child's difficulties, which makes it impossible to intelligently discuss the goals and targets of intervention.

Second, the emphasis of our formulation is the child's *cognitive* difficulties, not his behavior. As described in Chapter 1 (and in greater detail in ensuing chapters), focusing on cognition helps caretakers identify and understand what they are actually trying to work on with the child and therefore also clarifies their role in intervention.

Third, as we mentioned earlier, by focusing on cognitive skills, adults now have a clearer sense about why motivational strategies have failed to satisfactorily address the child's difficulties. Reward-and-punishment programs don't effectively treat other learning disabilities—reading, writing, and arithmetic—and they don't effectively treat a learning disability in the domains of flexibility/adaptability, frustration tolerance, and problem solving either. In other words, reward-and-punishment programs do not train a child to shift cognitive set more readily, reflect upon how a problem has been solved previously, consider the likely outcomes of alternative solutions, enter a group competently, recognize that someone is sad, let other people know how he is feeling, or stay calm enough to think clearly. To reiterate, focusing on cognition helps adults move beyond popular motivational "explanations" for children's maladaptive behavior: "She's doing it for attention," "She's not motivated to do well," "She just wants control," "She just wants things her own way."

In fact, clinicians using the CPS model actively refute such explanations when they are proposed by suggesting alternative ways of conceptualizing the child's difficulties that (we believe) are not only more accurate but also more likely to lead to productive interventions. Early in treatment, the clinician may be a bit more tentative in suggesting these alternative explanations, with the aim of simply raising the possibility of another way of thinking about the child. Once a consensus has been achieved about the cognitive factors underlying a child's struggles with flexibility and frustration tolerance, however, it may be necessary to be a bit more assertive in countering "regression to the mean" (i.e., a return to habitual motivational explanations). Witness the examples provided below—first from an initial session and then from a typical session later in treatment with the same family:

First Session

THERAPIST: (*to parents*) So what's your feeling about why Kelly acts this way?

FATHER: I think it's pretty clear that she knows that she can get her way so long as she continues to push it—especially with her mother. I'm not as likely to give in, and I think she's also a little more intimidated by me. I mean, I can make her go to her room if I need to carry her.

THERAPIST: Well, from what you've told me so far, I'm not sure that that's the only explanation. In fact, it seems pretty clear that her difficult behavior causes her a lot more pain than pleasure.

FATHER: That's true, but my daughter is also one of the world's best manipulators.

THERAPIST: Actually, it's possible that she's a good manipulator, but if she's like most of the kids we see, it's actually pretty unlikely that she's very good at it.

MOHER: What do you mean?

THERAPIST: Well, I've heard from you guys and read from her teachers that she is a very disorganized, impulsive thinker, right? Competent manipulation requires organization, impulse control, planning . . . the best indicator of competent manipulation is that the person who's being manipulated doesn't know it!

FATHER: I see what you mean, but sometimes I'm still pretty sure that she's up to something!

THERAPIST: Again, we'll see, but so far I'm wondering whether it might be more accurate to say that something's up with Kelly rather than that she's up to something! As we'll talk about, how we explain her behavior has a lot to do with what we try to do to fix the problem.

Session 4

THERAPIST: So how are things going?

MOTHER: We had a tough weekend. I mean in general things are still going better, but she was just pushing our buttons and her sister's buttons every chance she got this weekend!

THERAPIST: We'll have to figure out why this was such a tough weekend. But I'm a little confused . . . I thought we had decided that button pushing is not what Kelly's about . . . and that she'd like nothing better than to have things go better at home. Did something happen to cause us to change who we think she is and why she behaves the way she does?

Notice that the therapist is not afraid to jump right in even though the session has just started. If the therapist allows old explanations to stand, then she is implicitly agreeing with a return to an incorrect and unhelpful conceptualization of the child's behavior.

MOTHER: Sorry, I didn't mean it that way.

THERAPIST: No need for an apology. I just want to make sure we stay on top of our explanations for Kelly's difficulties, because those explanations have a lot to do with how we respond to her. I think that when things get a little tough, it's easy for old explanations that have never served us well to find their way back into our thinking. Or maybe the idea that her behavior is intentional still lurks somewhere just beneath the surface. In the past, that way of thinking has led you to use a lot of punishment to try to give her the incentive to behave appropriately.

MOTHER: And that certainly hasn't worked!

THERAPIST: Right . . . that's because motivation isn't the problem. I think we've agreed that the problem is Kelly's rigid, inflexible style of thinking and her very disorganized, impulsive way of solving problems.

FATHER: Funny, that's exactly what happened yesterday. Her little sister came into the kitchen when Kelly was playing cards with her mom and said that she had a loose tooth. Of course, her little sister's only 3 and doesn't really have any loose teeth . . . she was just pretending. But Kelly couldn't handle it . . . she insisted that Bridget was lying and that she needed to be punished for not telling the truth. We tried to explain that Bridget was just pretending, but Kelly got all hot and bothered and started screaming and saying that we always take her sister's side with things.

THERAPIST: So this was another case of Kelly's concrete, literal thinking making things messy in a hurry?

MOTHER: And I bet telling her to leave her sister alone was not the right thing to do, huh? (*laughter*)

THERAPIST: Well, it would make sense for kids who don't have Kelly's difficulties. But in Kelly's case, we're going to need a more specialized approach that would actually help us take those difficulties into account and, ultimately, fix them.

Again, perhaps most importantly, focusing on cognitive skills helps adults understand that explosive episodes are *highly predictable* and therefore permits a shift in the focus of intervention from consequences (reactively addressing the child's difficulties after the fact through motivational procedures) to *antecedents* (proactively addressing the child's difficulties before the fact by solving problems before they arise and teaching lacking thinking skills).

Let's go back to our first dialogue about Janet. We've established that many of Janet's explosive episodes (we think these might be better referred to as "incompatibility episodes") occur around homework. There's actually very little that can be done to prevent explosive episodes once Janet is upset about homework (again). Punishing Janet so as to give her the incentive not to get upset about her homework would make little sense because it wouldn't address the cognitive factors that are causing her to become upset about her homework in the first place. But there is a great deal that can be done to address these cognitive factors and solve the homework problem *before* Janet attempts another homework assignment, including remediation of the issues that are interfering with homework completion or making adjustments in the nature of homework assignments. This shift in mentality is further elucidated in upcoming chapters.

Q & A

What do you do when you're getting strong signals on a large number of items on the Pathways Inventory?

Many explosive kids have lagging cognitive skills in multiple domains. It won't be possible to address all lagging skills at once, and some skills require more time than others to remediate. Adult caretakers will need guidance in prioritizing and organizing their efforts, so "triage" is a very important function for the therapist. Unfortunately, we can't offer a prioritization algorithm; triage tends to be a matter of clinical judgment. As discussed in Chapter 6, in some instances the priority is on training skills required for the child and adult to participate in collaborative problem-solving discussions. In other cases, the priority is on addressing the lagging skills or triggers that are most destabilizing or accounting for a significant percentage of explosive episodes. Sometimes stability can be dramatically improved simply by addressing a high-potency or high-frequency trigger (e.g., homework). Sometimes the clinician discovers that many triggers (e.g., arguing with parents, fighting with siblings, bossing peers) trace back to a single lagging skill (e.g., not appreciating the impact of one's behavior on others); in these cases, teaching that skill might take priority because many triggers will be resolved by doing so. Once skills and triggers of the highest priority have been identified, others will naturally be placed on the "back burner" until the priorities have been addressed.

What do you do if you don't seem to get strong signals on any of the pathways?

Keep trying. Our data and experience tell us that some of the lacking cognitive skills contained within the pathways can be found in virtually all explosive kids. Sometimes caretakers are not especially astute observers of the factors that may have contributed to an explosive episode. As discussed earlier, we ask caretakers to tell us stories about explosive episodes, and we try to make sense of these stories by trying to identify lagging skills or triggers that would explain incompatibility under various circumstances. Of course, there is no substitute for what has been called the sine qua non of behavioral assessment: direct behavioral observation.

Are there times when factors other than lagging thinking skills can be important contributors to explosive episodes?

Yes. In those fairly rare instances when the pathways do not fully explain explosive episodes, we are on the lookout for (and routinely inquire about) other factors: sleep issues, current trauma, seizure disorders, food and seasonal allergies, drug or alcohol use, and other complicating medical conditions or reactions to medicine.

How do you know when to refer for formal testing?

We typically refer a child for neuropsychological assessment when interviews and observations don't provide enough definitive information to identify the specific skill deficits that are contributing to explosive episodes, or when we are interested in clarifying specific skills. We don't think every explosive child requires neuropsychological assessment. In many instances, we think it's possible to get a fairly good handle on pathways and triggers just by asking the right questions and through direct observation. On the other hand, there are certainly instances in which we felt we had a reasonable grasp of a child's pathways early on and then—perhaps because response to treatment was not as rapid or positive as anticipated—return to the "drawing board" to explore the possibility that potential triggers and skills had been overlooked. In such instances, formal assessment can be quite helpful.

Chapter 3

Options for
Handling Problems

Three Plans

It's probably worthwhile to take a brief look at where we've been before we head further down the road. Focusing on lagging cognitive skills helps move intervention away from motivational explanations and toward understanding problematic interactions between a child and an adult, at least partially, as the by-product of a learning disability in the domains of flexibility/ adaptability, frustration tolerance, and problem solving. This focus also helps us to identify the specific cognitive skills requiring remediation and permits us to tailor treatment to the needs of each child and his or her caretakers. By emphasizing a transactional model and incompatibility, we are explicitly assuming that the child's lagging cognitive skills only partially explain his difficulties and that pathways and triggers may well have relevance to the interaction partners with whom explosive episodes occur. Finally, by highlighting situational specificity, we are underscoring the fact that incompatibilities fueling explosive episodes are highly predictable and can therefore often be addressed well in advance.

These considerations have been incorporated into a framework known previously as the three "baskets" (this term came from the early days of the CPS model in which it was felt that people might benefit from the visual metaphor of having three baskets in front of them and depositing different problems or unmet expectations into the baskets depending on how each was to be handled). What we now refer to as the "plans framework" has multifaceted applications, but we'll begin with the most basic: helping adults come to recognize their options for responding to problems or unmet expectations in their child and the manner by which these options affect both their relationship with the child and the child's behavior.

THREE PLANS

While there are myriad ways in which adults respond to problems or unmet expectations with children, the plans framework places these options into three basic categories. The first option, known as "Plan A," involves the imposition of adult will . . . in other words, adults insisting that their expectations be met. This is, of course, an extremely popular option. The second option, known as "Plan B," involves engaging the child in a collaborative process of problem solving so as to resolve whatever concerns or factors are interfering with expectations being met (this option is far less popular but happens to be the major focus of this book). The third option, "Plan C," involves reducing or removing expectations, at least temporarily (this is a fairly popular option as well). All three can be effective responses, depending on the needs and capabilities of each child and the goals of each adult. This simple framework is the mechanism by which we help adults begin to categorize and reflect upon their own behavior and reevaluate and prioritize expectations as we work toward the goals of solving problems, reducing explosive episodes, improving adult–child interactions, and training lacking cognitive skills.

By the way, one of the most common misinterpretations of the CPS model is the belief that the model requires adults to *suspend* all of their expectations. So it is important to establish early on that the CPS model carries the assumption that *adults having expectations for children is a good thing*. Naturally, the degree to which various expectations are *realistic* is often an important focus of treatment. Thus, rather than reflecting some sort of hierarchy or ranking system, each plan represents distinct options for responding *when realistic expectations are not being met*. Let's consider Plan A and Plan C in greater detail (Chapter 4 is devoted entirely to Plan B).

Plan A

When a child does not meet expectations, it is very common for adults to insist more intensively. For example, if a child were not meeting the parental expectation of brushing his or her teeth at bedtime, Plan A would involve more intensive insistence that the child brush his or her teeth. Presumably, this insistence flows from the belief that the child failed to comprehend the importance or necessity of the expectation or perhaps needed a bit of a push. In ordinary children, this imposition of adult will does not typically have major adverse ramifications, both because the child does not have an extreme reaction to the intensive insistence and because the child ultimately meets the expectation (having now comprehended its importance or registered the meaning of the little extra push).

However, in the case of explosive children—due to any or many of the cognitive factors discussed in Chapter 1—imposition of adult will (Plan A) greatly *increases* the probability of an explosive episode and therefore does have major adverse ramifications. The problem with Plan A does not lie in the fact that adults are pursuing their expectations, especially if the expectations are realistic (with "realistic" meaning that the child is already capable of meeting the expectation on a *consistent* basis). *The problem with Plan A lies in the fact that adult expectations are being pursued in a manner that greatly heightens the likelihood of explosive outbursts in certain children.* In other words, from a transactional perspective, there is incompatibility between the characteristics of a given child and the manner in which adults are pursuing their expectations.

Many adults respond to this incompatibility by *further* intensifying their application of Plan A, often by offering incentives or threatening punishment, with the aim of giving children additional motivation to respond adaptively to Plan A. According to conventional wisdom, the child's poor response to Plan A is merely a learned means of forcing adults to relent or capitulate. The adults are understandably adverse to the prospect of "giving in" to the child. Since such a mentality is fairly ingrained in American culture (but less so, we have found, in some other cultures), we find that many adults who embrace this mentality have simply never given the matter much thought or have never been exposed to a cognitive perspective on children's behavior, and therefore do not have any alternative tools in their "discipline" repertoires. The CPS model provides adults with an opportunity to give the matter more thought and question these popular assumptions, expose adults to a cognitive perspective, and help adults (1) understand that there are actually *three* options for responding to problems or unmet expectations in children, (2) recognize that they have primarily been approaching such problems and unmet expectations with Plan A, and (3) recognize that one of the other two response options may actually be a better "fit" given the cognitive characteristics of their child.

Plan A is so habitual for many adults (including many clinicians), and so much an established and valued part of our culture, that many adults aren't even aware of when they are using Plan A. Thus, we often find that we need to provide adults with guidance to help them recognize when they are imposing their will or assuming a posture that is inherently inflexible. The following are common Plan A entry phrases: "No," "You must," You can't," and "1 . . . 2 . . . 3. . . . " In contrast to some other therapeutic modalities, *the CPS approach places no emphasis on teaching adults to execute Plan A proficiently.* Indeed, the CPS model actively aims to help adults address problems and pursue their expectations by using Plan B rather than Plan A.

Plan C

Plan C, once again, involves reducing or removing a given expectation. Plan C is highly effective at reducing a child's global level of frustration. Adults signal that they are using Plan C when they say nothing or simply convey that they do not object to a child's request or behavior (e.g., "OK"). For example, in the case of a child who is balking at brushing his teeth, Plan C would typically involve dropping the demand altogether. Note that when adults employ Plan C, the goal of reducing the likelihood of an explosive episode is achieved. However, also note that the goal of pursuing what one perceives to be an important adult expectation (the brushing of teeth) is not achieved.

We're never sure how adults are going to respond to our suggestion that some expectations be handled using Plan C. Some are relieved that someone official is giving them permission to reduce or eliminate expectations about which they themselves may have had reservations. Others fear that using Plan C means that the expectation will *never* be met (in the case of teeth brushing, this fear legitimately conjures up images of massive dental bills or toothless children). We frequently find that adults need some reassurance on the point that most of the realistic expectations temporarily being placed on the "back burner" early in treatment will find their way back into our discussions once a child's difficulties are well understood and family stability improved.

Let it be said that, under ordinary circumstances, teeth brushing is a perfectly legitimate expectation. One would not begin to ponder the importance of this expectation, and how it should be handled if unmet, unless one arrived at the conclusion that (1) there may be valid (perhaps motoric, sensory, or mood) issues interfering with the child brushing his teeth, or (2) the child is so impaired in the domains of flexibility and frustration tolerance that, at the end of a long day, adding one more demand or frustration to the mix breaks the proverbial camel's back.

Many adults unfamiliar with the CPS model rapidly define Plan C as "giving in." Actually, the definition of "giving in" is when an adult begins handling an expectation using Plan A and then winds up using Plan C because of the child's unpleasant response. When an adult *begins* with Plan C, the adult is merely indicating they have no expectation or concern, or that an expectation is not presently being pursued, perhaps because other expectations are higher in the hierarchy or because, given a clearer understanding of a child's difficulties, the expectation is now deemed to be unrealistic. Other adults confuse Plan C with "ignoring." The two terms are not synonymous. When employed as a behavior management tool, ignoring represents an effort to withdraw adult attention to or reinforcement for a given behavior. Once again, Plan C simply means that an adult is choosing not to pursue a given expectation.

GOALS OF INTERVENTION

With Plan B adults are attempting to engage the child in a process of working toward a mutually satisfactory resolution of adult and child concerns. We're going to forego discussion of this option—at least until the next chapter—in favor of highlighting several important points.

Because the CPS model was originally developed for the treatment of very difficult children and adolescents, the model delineates three basic goals of intervention. One goal is to dramatically *reduce the frequency, intensity, and duration of explosive episodes*. This goal can be achieved by handling many adult expectations with Plan C (explosive episodes should reduce in frequency if the expectations that were causing the outbursts are reduced or eliminated, and perhaps even in intensity as the general level of frustration in child and adult subsides). When certain pathways (primarily emotion regulation and executive skills) are involved, psychotropic medication may also be useful for achieving this goal (we think psychotropic medication is most likely to be overutilized when Plan C is underutilized and cognitive pathways are neglected). Plan B is also highly effective at reducing explosive episodes. By contrast, Plan A tends to precipitate explosive episodes.

A second goal of intervention is to help adults *pursue expectations*. Two Plans (A and B) can achieve this goal. With Plan A, adults are pursuing their expectations by imposing their will, often at the cost of inducing an explosive episode. Adults are also pursuing their expectations with Plan B, but instead of imposing their will to accomplish the mission, they are instead engaging the child in a collaborative effort to reach a mutually satisfactory solution to the problems interfering with expectations being met. The exact same expectation that can be pursued with Plan A can also be pursued with Plan B.

A third goal of intervention is to *teach cognitive skills that are lacking.* Neither Plan A nor Plan C is effective in achieving this goal. In other words, the cognitive deficits encompassed by the pathways are not effectively trained through either imposition of adult will or elimination of adult expectations. As described in the next chapter, Plan B is a highly effective means of teaching such skills. Indeed, as depicted in the graphic below, it is only Plan B that helps us achieve all three goals of intervention simultaneously: reduced explosive episodes, pursuit of adult expectations, and the teaching of lacking cognitive skills. Thus, successful implementation of Plan B—that is, helping adults and children engage in collaborative problem solving—is essential.

Goals Achieved by Each Plan

	Pursue expectations	Reduce outbursts	Teach skills
Plan A	√		
Plan C		√	
Plan B	√	√	√

Many adults overemphasize Plan A (imposition of will) prior to and early in treatment because they have yet to recognize the limitations imposed on their child by the pathways (in other words, they do not yet understand that Plan A is not well matched to their child's characteristics and needs). These adults tend to be quite focused on the legitimacy of their expectations and the future adverse ramifications on the child's development and long-term outcome if these expectations are abandoned. Typically, such adults are causing and enduring a lot of explosive episodes. These adults can be reassured on the legitimacy of their concerns ("Yes, it is important that Juan brush his teeth"), but encouraged to begin pondering whether (1) the expectation is realistic at this point in the child's development, or (2) whether there might be ways to pursue the expectation in a manner that does not cause explosive outbursts.

Overreliance on Plan A can also stem from the common misimpression that Plan A is a more efficient or faster way to pursue expectations. After all, why have a discussion with a child when you can just tell him what to do? Indeed, Plan A is quicker on the *front end* (it is far easier to just say no than it is to try to collaborate on solutions). But Plan B is more efficient on the *back end* and over the *long haul*—that is, the time spent problem solving together is generally far less than what is required in dealing with a child who has spiraled out of control and become violent or destructive. In other words, explosive episodes (precipitated by Plan A) always consume more time than solving problems durably. And unsolved problems are, of course, far more time-consuming than solved problems.

In some cases, of course, adult expectations are unrealistic and require examination. Discussions along these lines focus on whether a child's capacity to meet specific expectations is being compromised by his cognitive skill deficits. For example, let's say that we have established that shifting cognitive set is an area of vulnerability for a child. Let's say that we have also found (through our situational analysis) that a child has frequent explosive episodes during weekends. Upon further inquiry, let's say that we have learned that the child's weekend schedule is configured in a way that requires frequent shifting from one activity to another. Discussions can now center on (1) the fact that the schedule and the child's cognitive skills are poorly matched, (2) the fact that adult insistence (Plan A) is not improving the child's capacity for set shifting (but is causing many explosive episodes), and (3) that there might be a better way to pursue adult expectations without placing cognitive demands upon the child that he is currently unable to meet.

In the case of highly unstable children, the discussion about unrealistic expectations focuses less on specific cognitive skills and more on the child's general level of functioning. The goal of these discussions is to handle most expectations with Plan C, at least temporarily: "I think that under ordinary circumstances clean teeth is a reasonable expectation . . . but we are not currently operating under ordinary circumstances. I think that our most important focus at the moment is to help Billy become more stable so we don't have to admit him to an inpatient unit. So I'm thinking we might want to forego clean teeth for the time being so we don't cause unnecessary explosive episodes over things that aren't as crucial as they might seem under more stable circumstances. Once he stabilizes, we'll get back to clean teeth."

Adults who overemphasize Plan C (dropping or reducing expectations) may or may not understand the child's limitations but are quite clear about their desire to avoid explosive episodes. Such adults are probably enduring fewer explosive episodes but, having eliminated their expectations, may feel guilty and powerless. Others may energetically advocate for others to follow suit in reducing or dropping expectations, drawing criticism for having abdicated their adult responsibilities and capitulated to the child's wishes. Of course, adults who are overemphasizing Plan C still face the same dilemma as those overemphasizing Plan A: how to pursue expectations without causing explosive outbursts.

Many adults end up sitting on both sides of the fence: they employ Plan A (and endure explosive episodes) in pursuing the expectations they feel are most important and use Plan C (and avoid explosive episodes) to dispense with expectations they feel are least important or when the child responds explosively to Plan A. Seldom do adults find this "picking your battles" state of affairs to be satisfactory, for their approach to discipline has been reduced to the unpleasant task of deciding whether pursuing specific expectations is worth the price of an explosive episode.

In many two-parent families, of course, one parent overemphasizes Plan A while the other overemphasizes Plan C. These parents, too, find their situation to be unsatisfactory, for while there is the façade of "balance" in such a scenario, the parents have yet to agree upon who their child is and what his capabilities are, and therefore whether to pursue specific expectations. Such parents argue frequently with each other; the "Plan A parent" typically accuses the "Plan C parent" of being passive and permissive, and the "Plan C parent" commonly accuses the "Plan A parent" of being overly aggressive and harsh. Of course, helping both parents execute Plan B more proficiently is likely to achieve a healthier, more unified balance and simultaneously address the incompatibilities that are giving rise to explosive episodes in the first place. Plan B is not the "average" of Plans A and C.

It should be obvious that while Plan C may be of significant importance early in treatment, especially with highly unstable children, ultimately Plan A and Plan C are both of extremely limited utility in the CPS treatment framework. After a few quick questions, we'll turn to a more comprehensive discussion of the response category on which the success of CPS hinges: Plan B.

Q & A

I'm a little confused. If you're not using Plan A, how does the child know you have an expectation?

This question highlights one of the main ways in which the CPS model is often misinterpreted, in that a lot of adults make the mistake of believing that if they simply *have* an expectation, then they must be using Plan A. In fact, the plans aren't even a consideration until an expectation isn't being met. If a child is brushing his teeth as often and as well as his parents would like, that's a *met* expectation, and the plans aren't needed. If child is doing his homework as well and as reliably as his teachers would like, that's a *met* expectation, and the plans aren't needed. But if a child isn't meeting expectations for brushing teeth, or doing homework, or doing chores, or getting along with his classmates or siblings, those are *unmet* expectations, and now you have three options: with Plan A you're imposing your will, with Plan C you're dropping the expectation, and with Plan B you're collaboratively solving the problems and teaching the lacking skills that are interfering with the expectation being met.

Of course, how one informs (or reminds) a child of an expectation can cause an explosive outburst before one has the chance to use any plan. Tone will be an important issue here but, as you might imagine, "Get your butt in that kitchen and do the dishes" would be a fairly inflammatory way to express an expectation, whereas "Don't forget about the dishes" would be closer to the mark.

I just want to make sure I'm clear about something. If you're using Plan C, you're not applying it universally but only on certain problems or triggers, right?

Right. You'll be using Plan C on some triggers, Plan B on others.

So it's really possible to address unmet expectations and solve problems without using Plan A?

Not just possible . . . probable. But there's more to it than you've read so far.

Chapter 4

Plan B Basics

Here's what you already know: Plan A is a way to pursue expectations with a child, but (in the case of some children) often at the expense of an explosive episode. Plan C is a way to reduce explosive episodes, but at the expense of eliminating or reducing a given adult expectation (at least temporarily). And Plan B is a way to pursue adult expectations and resolve problems in a manner that is unlikely to cause an explosive episode while simultaneously teaching lacking cognitive skills. It may be obvious that, from our perspective, the key to successful treatment—and also the greatest challenge for clinicians—is helping adults and children productively interact and solve problems by using Plan B. Neither Plan A or Plan C teaches lagging cognitive skills. An important point to reiterate before we get started: Most adults won't appreciate the necessity of Plan B if they are not first aware of the lagging cognitive skills contributing to explosive episodes and of the fact that Plan A precipitates most of these episodes. In their eagerness to provide explicit guidance on implementation of the plans, clinicians often bypass the most important part: helping adult caretakes understand explosive episodes through the lens of triggers and pathways.

SURROGATE FRONTAL LOBE

When introducing Plan B, we often find it useful to tell adults that their role in Plan B is that of *surrogate frontal lobe*. This terminology makes explicit the fact that, in using Plan B, adults are going to do the thinking for a child that (at this point in his development) he is unable to do for himself. In the role of surrogate frontal lobe adults are accomplishing several very important missions: (1) walking the child through a frustrating situation in the present (and thereby preventing explosive episodes in the present); (2) solving problems routinely precipitating explosive episodes, preferably in a durable way; and (3) after multiple Plan B repetitions, training lacking thinking skills so that the child won't need a surrogate frontal lobe for the rest of his life.

"Surrogate frontal lobe" may not be familiar terminology for many adults (clinicians included), but adults commonly play this role in the lives of children. An adult is a surrogate frontal lobe when instructing a child on how to hit a baseball, teaching a child to read, providing guidance to a child on why it's generally not a good idea to cross the street without looking both ways, or helping an adolescent learn how to drive a car. In the case of explosive children, the surrogate frontal lobe is modeling and teaching the crucial skills of flexibility, frustration tolerance, and problem solving (along with some additional skills we'll get to in later chapters). Note that the manner in which Plan B is described below is very similar to the way we would describe Plan B to the adults with whom we work.

EMERGENCY PLAN B VERSUS PROACTIVE PLAN B

As we discussed in Chapter 2, explosive episodes occur only under certain conditions and are therefore highly predictable. In other words, we find that, within individual children and their families, these outbursts tend to occur repetitively in response to the same circumscribed sets of problems or triggers. Once again, this scenario has the potential to make resolution of these problems significantly easier, but for one unfortunate fact: most adults don't think about problems in situational terms, so they don't realize that the outbursts are highly predictable. Thus, many adults wait until they are in the throes of a (highly predictable) problem before attempting a Plan B dialogue. We refer to this as "Emergency Plan B" and, because of the heightened emotions characteristic of such moments, this is the least opportune time to attempt to durably solve a problem. This use of Plan B can be productive as a crisis-intervention or de-escalation tool. But because explosive episodes are highly predictable, the vast majority of Plan B discussions should be taking place *proactively*, well in advance. We call this "Proactive Plan B." It is the therapist's job to identify triggers that precipitate explosive episodes on a routine basis and help adults and children begin to have Proactive Plan B discussions under controlled circumstances (i.e., in the therapist's office) so that, over time, adults feel more confident about having these discussions without the therapist's assistance. So as you're reading about Plan B, resist the temptation to think of Plan B as what one does *once an explosive episode is set in motion; think of Plan B as how one solves a problem before it arises yet again.*

RUDIMENTARY PLAN B

Several ingredients are necessary for individuals to successfully collaborate on solutions to problems or disagreements. First, it is important for both parties to remain calm so that rational discourse can take place. Second, it is important to ensure that the concerns of both parties are clearly defined and entered into consideration. Third, it is crucial to entertain the wide range of possible solutions that could address both sets of concerns.

These ingredients are incorporated into the three steps necessary for successful execution of Plan B:

1. *Empathy (plus reassurance)*
2. *Define the problem*
3. *Invitation*

We tell adults that the only way they can be certain that they are doing Plan B is to use the three steps in the proper sequence. If they don't use the three steps in the prescribed sequence, they're not doing Plan B.

Step 1: Empathy

Empathy is the first step for initiating Plan B for several very important reasons. First, Carl Rogers was right: feeling heard helps people feel understood and, if some other ingredients also fall into place, also *keeps people calm*. Second—and this is crucial—empathy acknowledges that the child has a legitimate concern and *defines that concern*. We think that adults are notorious for failing to acknowledge children's legitimate concerns and, even when such concerns are briefly acknowledged, minimizing their importance and supplanting them with adult concerns. Such a practice, of course, typically plants adults squarely in Plan A territory and teaches children that their concerns don't matter or, at the very least, haven't achieved the same level of importance or legitimacy as adult concerns. It's worth pondering whether this is actually the consistent message we want to be transmitting to someone we hope will be an adaptive, thinking adult someday.

Many adults need to be provided with specific modeling on how to empathize. A good rule of thumb for initiating empathy using Proactive Plan B is to begin with the words, "I've noticed that . . . ." With Emergency Plan B, empathy takes the form of reflective listening (i.e., an approximation or restatement of the child's concern). If our situational analysis has identified homework completion as a common precipitant for explosive episodes, at a very basic level empathy (using Proactive Plan B) might sound as follows: "I've noticed that homework has been a bit of a struggle lately, and I know that's no fun for you." If our situational analysis has instead determined that application of eczema cream at bedtime frequently precipitates explosive episodes, basic empathy (using Proactive Plan B) might sound as follows: "I've noticed that you're not very happy about having us put skin cream on you at night." And if our situational analysis has helped us recognize that snacking before mealtime is the cause of many explosive episodes, basic empathy (using Proactive Plan B) might sound like this: "I've noticed that you sometimes get very hungry before dinner."

This very basic form of empathy is only sometimes effective at ensuring that a child's concern has been identified and articulated. For example, "I've noticed that you sometimes get very hungry before dinner" is probably sufficient for defining the child's concern. But in the case of the first two examples—"I've noticed that homework has been a bit of a struggle lately, and I know that's no fun for you" and "I've noticed that you're not very happy about having us put skin cream on you at night"—we've not yet clarified the child's concern in a way that is specific enough to set the stage for problem solving. *Coming to a highly specific definition of the child's concern is absolutely essential.* Thus, there's more work to be done. Clarifying the child's concern usually involves asking a simple question after the initial stab at empathy: "What's up?" There are a variety of concerns that might be interfering with homework completion, including "It's too hard," "I can't write that much," "There's too much," "I'm too tired by then," "I don't understand what I'm supposed to do," "There's too much noise in the house," and so forth. Now *these* are problems that can be solved. *So long as the child's concern is poorly specified, the problem will not get solved.*

Along these lines, many children make their concerns known through pronouncements rather than by defining a specific problem. "I'm not taking my medicine" and "I'm not going to school" would be common examples. These statements would qualify more as *solutions* than as *concerns*. Once again, it will be necessary for adults to help the child be more specific about his concerns. After empathizing with these statements ("You're not taking your medicine" or "You're not going to school"), the clarification process begins by asking, "What's up?" In the case of the first statement, answers might include "It tastes bad," or "It makes me dizzy," or "I can't swallow the pill," or "It's making me fat." Once again, *these* are problems for which there may be any of a variety of solutions, but not if we get sidetracked by the statement "I'm not taking my meds." As regards the second pronouncement ("I'm not going to school"), responses to "What's up?" might include "Nobody likes me," "Mrs. Johnson gets mad when I don't understand something," or "The boys bother me on the playground." Again, these clarifications move us closer to solving actual problems than the original pronouncement. Indeed, often adults enter Plan B dialogues with certain assumptions about the child's concerns, only to have to shift gears when it turns out that the assumptions were completely off-base. It's no tragedy to have preconceived notions about a child's concern; adults must simply be open to the possibility that their preconceived notions are wrong! In Chapter 6, we provide details on what to do if a child is unable to identify or articulate his concerns.

Adults often have difficulty with this first step of Plan B, some because they fear that empathy is a sign that they're about to capitulate to the child's wishes, others because they just haven't had a lot of practice. Here are some examples of empathy (using Emergency Plan B) gone awry:

CHILD: I'm not doing my homework.

ADULT: (*attempted empathy, using Emergency B*) I didn't like doing my homework when I was your age either.

Here the adult is assuming that letting the child know you feel the same way or have had a similar experience qualifies as empathy. It doesn't. In fact, the net effect may actually be to minimize the child's concern, which, it's worth noting, is still ill-defined.

Another example:

CHILD: I want pizza.

ADULT: (*empathy, using Emergency B*) You must be very hungry.

Believe it or not, here the adult has taken a bit of a leap in the empathy department. While there's some chance the adult is correct, in some children there
can be a big price to be paid for being wrong: an explosive episode. Indeed, in
the midst of frustration, some children don't have the wherewithal (often, but
not always, linguistic) to correct well-intentioned but misguided empathy. In
such cases, we think it makes more sense strategically to stick with basic, "low-
risk" empathy and to ask the child to define his concern. Once the concern has
been more clearly defined, the adult should reempathize. If the child can't define the concern, the adult can begin making educated guesses. Here are two
examples:

CHILD: I want pizza.

ADULT: (*empathy, using Emergency B*) You want pizza. What's up?

CHILD: You said we could have pizza today!

ADULT: (*reempathizing*) I said we could have pizza today.

*   *   *

CHILD: I'm not taking my meds.

ADULT: (*empathy, using Emergency B*) You're not taking your meds. What's
    up?

CHILD: I don't know!

ADULT: Should we try to figure it out?

CHILD: Fine!

ADULT: Well, I've noticed that you sometimes have trouble swallowing the
    pill. Is that it?

CHILD: No!

ADULT: Is it that you don't like the way it tastes on your tongue?

CHILD: Yes!

ADULT: (*reempathizing*) You don't like the way the medicine tastes on your
    tongue.

In some instances, empathy does not keep a child calm because adults
use it to segue into Plan A:

ADULT: (*using Proactive B, but only momentarily*) I've noticed that you some-
    times get very hungry before dinner is on the table . . . (*here's the segue
    into A*) but you're just going to have to wait.

This, of course, is the worst possible use of empathy because it fairly rapidly causes the child to lose faith that empathy is the starting signal for Plan B.

Some children may be so accustomed to adults handling problems or unmet expectations with Plan A that mere empathy is not a strong enough signal that the adults are taking a different tack. In other cases, the child's affective response to frustration may be so abrupt and intense that additional calming is needed. In both scenarios, a bit of *reassurance* is sometimes necessary— reassurance, that is, that the adult is not doing Plan A (e.g., "I'm not saying no" or "I'm not saying you have to"). Here's what this would sound like:

ADULT: (*empathy, using Proactive B*) I've noticed that homework has been a struggle lately. What's up?

CHILD: I don't want to do it right after school.

ADULT: (*reempathizing*) You don't want to do it right after school. How come?

CHILD: Because I'm tired . . . I need a break.

ADULT: (*reempathizing*) Let me make sure I've got this right . . . you don't want to do your homework right after school because you're tired and you need a break. Yes?

CHILD: Right!

ADULT: (*reassurance*) I'm not saying you have to do your homework right after school.

Of course, the adult isn't saying the child *doesn't* have to do the homework right after school, either. The important thing about empathy is that it's neither an indication of agreement nor disagreement . . . neither a "yes" nor a "no" . . . but merely a way to keep the child (and adult) calm and ensure that the child's concern (e.g., fatigue after school) is entered into consideration.

It is also important to recognize that using Plan B words with an angry, accusatory, condescending, or belittling tone won't get the job done. And Plan A can be executed in a soft, gentle tone—we call this "Gentle A" or "Soft A"—but it's still Plan A, and the child's reaction is likely be about the same as with "harder" forms of Plan A.

We have come to realize that most humans greatly overestimate their skills at empathy or simply don't see the point. Naturally, if an adult is having difficulty empathizing with a child's concerns, it is the therapist's role to teach the skill. More on this topic later in this chapter.

Step 2: Define the Problem

Once the child's concern has been acknowledged and defined, it is time for the second step of Plan B: define the problem. This is the step in which adults enter *their* concerns into consideration. This is a crucial step, for if there aren't two concerns on the table there is little likelihood that two interaction partners are actually in a position to solve a given problem collaboratively. In other words, if there's only one concern on the table and it's the *Adult's* concern, that's Plan A. And if there's only one concern on the table and it's the *Child's* concern, that's Plan C. There's only one plan in which *Both* concerns are on the table: Plan B. That's why this step is called "define the problem"—because *the definition of a problem is simply two concerns that have yet to be reconciled*.

Adults often announce their concerns through pronouncements (solutions) in the same way that children do: "You're not having a snack because it will spoil your dinner!" or "We're putting your eczema cream on before bedtime because I don't feel like dealing with you scratching all night!" or "You're doing homework right after school because that's the best time!" As we've already suggested, these pronouncements are sometimes a sign that adults feel that their concerns take precedence over children's concerns. Of course, adults who evidence this mind-set will probably need to be helped to appreciate the legitimacy of children's concerns (return to empathy) or to be educated about the pathways that are interfering with their child responding in an adaptive manner to Plan A. In other instances, pronouncements are a sign of adults' fears that their concerns won't be heard or taken into account (Plan A ensures that this fear is passed from one generation to the next). Therapists can help such adults understand that their concerns will be heard and taken into account with Plan B. *But Plan B cannot move forward if the adults' concerns are poorly specified.*

We often find that such pronouncements are a sign that adults don't really know what their concerns are. In such instances, the therapist's role is to help clarify the adults' concerns by asking a very important question: *"What's your concern about that?"* For example, "What's your concern about Stephanie having a snack before dinner?" or "Why does Ezra need to put the eczema cream on at bedtime?" In the case of the first question, the most likely answer would be "I didn't want him to spoil his dinner," but could conceivably include something like "I didn't have a problem with him eating something before dinner, but I wanted it to be something healthy." Now, *these* are concerns for which there might be a variety of solutions. In the case of the second question, possible concerns would include "I hate to see him be so itchy all night" or "If we don't stay on top of the eczema he'll have to take medicine orally, and he hates pills." Once again, these are valid concerns, but the child won't have the opportunity to take these concerns into account and collaborate on mutually satisfactory courses of action unless the adults' concerns are well specified. One of the crucial roles of the therapist is helping adults recognize the difference between solutions and concerns.

By the way, it is sometimes the case that adults discover they really don't have a concern to put on the table. That means the child's concern is the only concern on the table, and that means the problem is now being handled with Plan C:

ADULT: My son won't come home for lunch when he's playing at a friend's house.

THERAPIST: How have you been handling that problem?

ADULT: I've been demanding that he come home for lunch at 1:00 P.M. That's Plan A, right?

THERAPIST: Right. How's that approach been working?

ADULT: He goes ballistic.

THERAPIST: What's your concern about him not coming home for lunch?

ADULT: You know, as we're talking, I'm starting to wonder about that. I mean, what's gonna happen? It's not like he's gonna starve!

THERAPIST: Unless there's something you haven't told me about him, you're probably right.

ADULT: So maybe I don't really have a concern?

THERAPIST: Maybe not.

ADULT: So that's Plan C, right?

THERAPIST: Right.

ADULT: You mean I've been causing all these explosions when I didn't even have a concern?

Here's how Plan B sounds with the Define the Problem step now added:

ADULT: (*empathy, using Proactive B*) I've noticed that homework has been a struggle lately. What's up?

CHILD: I don't want to do it right after school.

ADULT: (*reempathizing*) You don't want to do it right after school. How come?

CHILD: Because I'm tired . . . I need a break.

ADULT: (*reempathizing*) Let me make sure I've got this right . . . you don't want to do your homework right after school because you're tired and you need a break. Yes?

CHILD: Right!

ADULT: (*reassurance and defining the problem*) I'm not saying you have to do your homework right after school, and I definitely don't want to keep fighting with you about it. But I'm very concerned that if you don't do it right after school it won't get done.

Step 3: Invitation

The third step of Plan B involves *inviting* the child to collaboratively brainstorm ideas for solving the problem in a way that is *feasible* and *mutually satisfactory*. The invitation makes it clear that solving the problem is something child and adult are doing together. The key word in initiating the invitation is "let's"—as in, "Let's think about how we can solve that problem," or "Let's see if we can figure that out," or "Let's see what we can do about that"—although many kids (and adults) find it helpful for the concerns of both parties to be restated as part of the invitation so as to summarize the problem that is to be solved (e.g., "Let's think about how we can make sure you get your homework done without your having to do it right after school").

It is at this point that child and adult brainstorm solutions that would address both of the concerns that have now been entered into discussion. We typically recommend that the child be given the first crack at generating solutions (usually by saying something along the lines of "Do you have any ideas?"), but this doesn't mean the burden is upon the child to solve the problem. The burden is upon both members (child and adult) of the problem-solving team to solve the problem, and it doesn't matter whose solution is ultimately selected. What matters is that the solution be *feasible and mutually satisfactory*. There is no such thing as a bad solution—only solutions that aren't feasible or mutually satisfactory. So, if in response to "Do you have any ideas?" a child says "No," the adult might respond, "Well, I have a few ideas . . . would you like to hear them?" If the child responds with a solution that isn't feasible (for either of the two parties), the adult might respond, "Well, there's an idea . . . but as I think about it, I'm not sure I (or you) can actually do my (or your) part a lot of the time . . . let's think of a solution that we both can actually do." Or, if the child responds with a solution that would not be mutually satisfactory, the adult might respond,

"Well, that solution would probably work well for you but it wouldn't work well for me. Let's try to think of a solution that would work well for both of us." At this point it would make sense to restate the two concerns to ensure that the participants haven't lost track of what problem they're trying to solve.

As you might expect, this third step presents another opportunity for the Plan B ship to run aground. For example, we work with many adults who, after having mastered the first two steps of Plan B (empathy and define the problem), still end up doing Plan A because they neglect to invite the child to solve the problem collaboratively. Often this is because the adults would never imagine that a child might have something to offer in the problem-solving department (this notion can usually be disproved fairly rapidly), or because the adult already has a solution formulated and can't adjust his or her original vision of how the problem should be solved (this scenario may require examination of adult pathways), or because Plan A is just a bad habit (practice makes perfect). In other instances, neither child nor adult has exceptional solution-generating skills. Or the child and adult may agree to a solution that is completely unrealistic. As discussed in Chapter 6, the therapist's role is to identify and articulate these issues and help steer the Plan B ship until child and adult are able to resolve problems independently and realistically. However, in its simplest form, here's how Plan B would sound using the three steps:

ADULT: (*empathy, using Proactive B*) I've noticed that homework has been a struggle lately. What's up?

CHILD: I don't want to do it right after school.

ADULT: (*reempathizing*) You don't want to do it right after school. How come?

CHILD: Because I'm tired . . . I need a break.

ADULT: (*reempathizing*) Let me make sure I've got this right . . . you don't want to do your homework right after school because you're tired and you need a break. Yes?

CHILD: Right!

ADULT: (*reassurance, defining the problem, and invitation*) I'm not saying you have to do your homework right after school, and I definitely don't want to keep fighting with you about it. But I'm very worried that if you don't do it right after school it won't get done. Let's think about how we can solve that problem.

EASY LIVING WITH PLAN B

Having now provided a general overview of rudimentary Plan B, let's examine how we might begin to weave Plan B into therapy and begin to consider the problems we are likely to encounter as we do so. Recall that prior to explaining Plan B to a child's caretakers, we've already discussed the pathways (skills that need to be trained) that may be interfering with the child's capacity for flexibility, frustration tolerance, and problem solving, and identified triggers (problems that have yet to be solved) that commonly precipitate explosive episodes. We have also tried to achieve an informal sense of the caretakers' capacities to digest and absorb this alternative view of the child's difficulties. As mentioned earlier, we do not have caretakers plunge into Plan B without first ensuring that they understand why it is crucial to teach lacking thinking skills and collaborate on solutions to problems, and why consequence-based programs are unlikely to accomplish these goals. But there are other issues that we may need to attend to before moving forward. What is the general level of stress in the caretakers? Will mere implementation of Plan B reduce the stress, or are other interventions (e.g., adjunctive therapies) indicated? Are there factors that may interfere with the adults' ability to successfully execute Plan B? If so, can we address these factors proactively? Is the child's level of hyperactivity or irritability or inability to tolerate frustration so extreme that we are dubious about his capacity to participate in Plan B discussions without pharmacological intervention? Is the level of hostility between the child and adult caretakers so extreme that it is not yet possible for them to participate in Plan B discussions, even with the therapist serving as mediator? Is the level of hostility or unsafe behavior so severe that more extreme measures must be taken (e.g., hospitalization, referral to protective services)? Do child and adult seem to possess the requisite skills for executing the three steps of Plan B?

Obviously, there are a variety of issues that could interfere with implementation of Plan B, and these issues are addressed in forthcoming chapters. Many readers might feel that the last issue—whether, in the clinician's judgment, child and adult have the skills to participate in Plan B discussions—is of particular importance. There's no question that in many cases some basic skills—identifying and articulating one's concerns, generating alternative solutions, considering the likely outcomes of solutions—must be trained prior to sending children and their adult caretakers out into the Plan B wilderness. We'll tackle this issue in Chapter 6.

Another consideration to be discussed more fully in later chapters is how best to utilize Plan B early in treatment. You see, Plan B can be utilized in two ways: for *resolving problems* or triggers (we call this *problem-focused Plan B*) and for *teaching lagging skills* (we call this *skill-focused Plan B*). If the clinician concludes that one or two key problems (e.g., homework and getting ready for school) are accounting for a meaningful percentage of explosive episodes, then early use of Plan B would be focused on resolving these problems (i.e., problem-focused Plan B). By contrast, if the clinician believes that many explosive episodes are precipitated by a particular lagging skill (e.g., difficulty appreciating how one's behavior is affecting others), then it might make sense to focus initial use of Plan B on teaching that skill (i.e., skill-focused Plan B).

Let's assume—at least, for the remainder of this chapter—that the clinician has concluded that the child and his adult caretakers are ready to take the Plan B plunge and that focusing on a few specific problems or triggers is the optimal way to utilize Plan B early in treatment. Our next step is to encourage adults to use Proactive Plan B to attempt to solve a few problems with the child prior to the next meeting and to keep a record of how things went. Once again, in assigning this homework, we are asking adults to focus on a few of the triggers—problems that have yet to be solved—that commonly precipitate explosive episodes.

In the next meeting, the adults are likely to report several instances in which Plan B was unsuccessful at producing a satisfactory outcome. This is usually expressed with the following statement: "Plan B isn't working." The role of the therapist is to figure out why. Below are some of the very common patterns to watch for and work on.

The Adults Used A When They Could Have Used B

Often adults who are new to Plan B feel that there are still many problems that they have no choice but to continue handling with Plan A. These problems provide an opportunity for the therapist to remind the adults that their concerns can be addressed with either Plan A or Plan B. Here's an example from a meeting with two parents:

MOTHER: There's one big issue we need to talk about today. From the minute Chris wakes up every day lately, all he wants to do is spend time with the kid next door, Jim. We don't mind him spending time with Jim, but we told him he has to have Jim over to our house. So whenever we tell him he can't go over to Jim's house, he starts to scream and yell and go crazy. Like this morning when he wanted to go over to Jim's house before the bus came, we said no, and he started throwing his backpack at us.

THERAPIST: (*clarifying the adult concern that led to Plan A in the first place*)

Why are you insisting that Chris and Jim play at your house instead of Jim's house? What's your concern about him playing at Jim's house?

MOTHER: Let's just say that Jim doesn't have the model family. Last week Jim's father and older brother got into a fistfight on the front lawn and the cops came. His father was put in jail for the night.

THERAPIST: So what you're saying is that you are very concerned about whether it's safe for Chris to play at Jim's house.

FATHER: You could say that!

THERAPIST: Sounds like a very legitimate concern. But remember, we have two options—Plan A and Plan B—for addressing your concerns. If you're using Plan A, Chris's concern is never acknowledged and there's no attempt to come up with a solution that he can live with. And, as you saw this morning, then he goes nuts. If we're doing Plan B, your concern still makes it onto the table but so does his concern. What are Chris's concerns?

The therapist's goal here is to help the parents understand that Plan A isn't their only option for solving problems . . . Plan B can get the job done as well (without the explosion). Of course, Plan B requires that their son's concern also make it into the discussion.

MOTHER: He wants to play with Jim all the time over at Jim's house.

THERAPIST: (*trying to ensure that the child's concern is on the table as well*) Any particular reason that Chris wants to play at Jim's house instead of your house?

FATHER: (*looks at wife*) You know, we've never really asked.

THERAPIST: So we don't really know why Chris is so invested in playing at Jim's house, or even if he is all that invested. This problem is currently being handled with Plan A. I'm wondering what this problem would look like if you were using Plan B.

MOTHER: Empathy first, right? We've got that part down. We'd tell him that we know he wants to play with Jim—and that he can as long as he plays with him at our house.

THERAPIST: Whoa. Be careful. I just heard you do empathy but then give him your solution. If you're doing Plan B, you're not solving the problem *for* him, you're solving it *with* him. Since we're not sure what his concern is, I think we'd want to ask the question "What's up?" Any ideas about what his answer would be?

FATHER: We have no idea. Maybe Jim has better video games than we do.

THERAPIST: OK, let's assume that's what he said. Let's go back to empathy because we've now clarified his concern.

MOTHER: OK. So I'd say, "You want to play at Jim's house because he has better video games than we do. Yes?"

THERAPIST: Great. Now your concern.

MOTHER: But we're very concerned that it's not safe at Jim's house.

FATHER: Yeah, but as soon as we say that he'll go nuts. He'd be throwing the backpack in a second.

THERAPIST: Well, you might be right about that, since staying calm in the midst of frustration isn't his strong suit. But we really won't know how he'll respond to Plan B until you actually do Plan B. You might want to reassure him that you're not using Plan A.

MOTHER: How?

THERAPIST: Well, just tell him that you're not saying he can't play at Jim's house.

FATHER: But we're not saying he can, right?

THERAPIST: That's right. But the reason he might go nuts on you is that he's anticipating that you're going to come forth with a flat-out no—Plan A. Of course, he's got a good reason—past history—for thinking that's what's going to happen. So we need to reassure him that that's not going to happen.

MOTHER: OK. So we tell him that he wants to play at Jim's house because Jim has better video games and that we're not saying no. Then we let him know that we need to know he's safe. Then what?

THERAPIST: Then you invite him to help work this out with you.

MOTHER: So what's the solution?

THERAPIST: Beats me. I suspect there are lots of solutions that would address both your concerns.

FATHER: Like playing at our house where we can keep an eye on him?

THERAPIST: That's one of many possible solutions.

FATHER: But isn't that where we started when he exploded this morning?

THERAPIST: Well, I must say, I'm not sure how exactly that particular solution would address Chris's concerns. Remember, the solution has to be mutually satisfactory. Also, I'm not even sure he heard your concern because it came in the form of a Plan A ultimatum. You just told him that he couldn't play at Jim's house, and he got upset. We never actually heard what he thought of that idea. In fact, it wasn't a discussion at all. It was just an ultimatum.

Here the therapist is reminding the parents of a few very important points. First, there is no such thing as *"the* solution." Plan B opens the discussion to a universe of possible solutions. Second, one of the most important aspects of a "good solution" is that it be mutually satisfactory . . . that is, that it address the concerns of both parties. Third, if there are two *solutions* on the table ("I want to play at Jim's house" and "You have to play at our house") rather than two *concerns*, then Plan B rapidly becomes mired in the mud of what we call "dueling solutions." When this happens, the therapist's role is to clarify the concerns of both parties so that collaborative problem solving can actually take place and to remind the participants of the difference between a concern and a solution.

FATHER: So Plan B is just a way to get him to do what we want without the explosion?

THERAPIST: Not exactly. If you already know what the solution is before you begin Plan B, you're not doing Plan B . . . you're doing Plan A. Don't forget, this is *collaborative* problem solving, not *unilateral* problem solving. The idea with Plan B is to work on the problem together and be open to any solution that you come up with as long as it addresses both concerns. In the process, Chris is learning how to work things out so he'll be better able to tolerate frustration the next time.

Another very important point is that a lot of adults enter Plan B discussions with very rigid ideas about the solution to the problem. But Plan B isn't *clever* Plan A. If adults wish to engage a child in a Plan B discussion, they must be open to different solutions for solving the problem.

FATHER: Well, the good news is that we'll have plenty of chance to practice since this issue comes up about 20 times a day lately. He's obsessed with playing with Jim.

THERAPIST: Well, you bring up another important point. This is a pretty predictable problem. In fact, we can predict that he will melt down several times a day if you're doing Plan A over playing at Jim's house. So this is a problem that we should be trying to solve before it becomes a problem.

MOTHER: How do you mean?

THERAPIST: Well, once Chris is begging you to play at Jim's house, he's already getting worked up and is probably not at his most rational.

FATHER: You got that right!

THERAPIST: So we should try to work this out with Chris when he's calm.

MOTHER: You mean bring it up before Chris does.

THERAPIST: Exactly . . . we call that Proactive Plan B. It saves you the trouble of doing Emergency Plan B over and over on the exact same issue.

MOTHER: We can try this.

THERAPIST: Just remember, this discussion can't take place unless Chris's concern is on the table and shouldn't take place if you guys already know what the solution is.

This dialogue demonstrates that it is possible for the therapist to empathize with an adult concern without endorsing a Plan A approach to its resolution.

Overreliance on Emergency Plan B

You've probably noticed that we've said precious little about Emergency Plan B to this point, and for good reason: we don't want people making Emergency Plan B a habit. It's there if people need it . . . if they are surprised by an explosive episode . . . if a new, unexpected trigger precipitated an explosive episode . . . if they are early in the Plan B implementation process and haven't quite pinpointed a child's pathways or triggers just yet.

Why are we less enthusiastic about Emergency Plan B? Again, because it has a lower likelihood of success than Proactive Plan B. Why? Again, because of added heat. It is the therapist's role to point out that problems that have been handled with Emergency Plan B can be resolved more productively— and more durably—with Proactive Plan B.

MOTHER: We nearly had an explosion on the way to your office.

THERAPIST: What happened?

MOTHER: Well, about 10 minutes before we got here, Izzy decided he was hungry. I think we actually handled it pretty well.

THERAPIST: Tell me.

MOTHER: Well, he's sitting in the back seat and we're cruising along and he announces that he wants pizza.

THERAPIST: Pizza?

MOTHER: Pizza.

THERAPIST: What did you say when he made that announcement?

MOTHER: I did the empathy thing . . . I said, "You want pizza."

THERAPIST: Of course, "I want pizza" isn't a very specific concern.

MOTHER: Right! So I said "What's up?" He said, "I'm hungry." So I said, "You're hungry."

THERAPIST: Great . . . what happened next?

MOTHER: Well, then I said what my concern was.

THERAPIST: What did you say?

MOTHER: I said I wanted to be on time for our appointment with you because I feel like I'm wasting money when we're late. Then I asked him if he had any ideas for how we could solve the problem.

THERAPIST: What did he say?

MOTHER: He started getting a little irritated. But he actually thought of a solution.

THERAPIST: He did? What was his solution?

MOTHER: He suggested that we stop at that gas station before your office and get some pretzels.

THERAPIST: Is that what you did?

MOTHER: Yes! And no explosion!

THERAPIST: Fabulous. Good for you. Now I have a question.

MOTHER: Uh-oh. I messed up.

THERAPIST: Nope, you did great. But I still have a question.

MOTHER: What's the question?

THERAPIST: How often does he get hungry in the car on the way to my office?

MOTHER: He always gets hungry in the car on the way to your office.

THERAPIST: That being the case . . . maybe we should try to solve this problem once and for all?

MOTHER: I don't understand what you mean.

THERAPIST: Well, we don't want you to have to do Emergency Plan B with him every time he gets hungry on the way to my office. I'm thinking this is a good opportunity to practice Proactive Plan B. Should we get him in here?

MOTHER: Sure.

THERAPIST: (*to child, now having joined the session*) I heard you did a great job in the car on the way here.

CHILD: Yup.

THERAPIST: You stayed calm and you and your mom solved the problem of you being hungry, yes?

CHILD: Yup.

THERAPIST: I've got another one for you.

CHILD: Another what?

THERAPIST: Another problem.

CHILD: OK.

THERAPIST: I understand that this isn't the first time you've gotten hungry in the car on the way to my office. Is that right?

CHILD: Yup.

THERAPIST: So I was saying to your mom that maybe we should get that problem solved once and for all.

CHILD: How?

THERAPIST: Well, let's think about it. You always get hungry on the way to my office. And your mom's always running late so she doesn't want to stop for food. Can you think of how you guys can work that out?

CHILD: Um . . . we could bring pretzels in the car with us.

THERAPIST: That's an idea. (*looking at mother*) Mom, what do you think of that idea?

MOTHER: I like it.

THERAPIST: (*to child*) That idea work for you, Izzy?

CHILD: Yup.

THERAPIST: You guys sure?

CHILD and MOTHER: Yup.

THERAPIST: Good. Sounds like the solution works for both of you. Is it do-able?

MOTHER: I don't see why not.

THERAPIST: If this solution works, then you guys won't have to keep solving the same problem over and over again week after week. In other words, this solution . . . if it works . . . should stand the test of time. What are you guys going to do if the solution stops working for some reason?

MOTHER: Talk about it again?

THERAPIST: Exactly. Preferably at opportune moments rather than when things are really hot.

Thus, when adults ask, "What should I do when he goes ballistic?" our response is, "Either Plan C or Emergency Plan B." Of course, the rejoinder is, "But then think about when you're going to have a Proactive Plan B discussion so you can get the problem that caused him to go ballistic solved once and for all." In other words, each explosive episode provides critical information about pathways or triggers we may have overlooked.

Indeed, it is often the case that the content of a Plan B discussion differs depending on whether one is utilizing Emergency versus Proactive B. For example, a little girl who was balking at going to the grocery store with her father after school identified as her concern that she wanted to go home first to visit with her dog. The Plan B discussion focused on taking this concern into account. But in the Proactive B discussion that followed—under much calmer conditions—the girl's concerns were that she found it boring at the grocery store and that her father never let her buy anything she wanted. The content of the ensuing discussion and the solutions under consideration were dramatically different, even though the trigger—going grocery shopping—was the same.

Adults and children can only have a finite number of Plan B discussions in one day. If the same issue requires fresh resolution on a daily basis—something we call *Perpetual Plan B*—then a lot of energy is being devoted to Plan B but the issue is not being durably resolved. Proactive Plan B should solve that problem.

Missing Steps

If Plan B isn't going well, there's an outstanding likelihood that adults are neglecting one of the three steps of Plan B. When adults announce at the beginning of a session that they tried to implement Plan B during the previous week and "it didn't work," our usual response is to ask that adults tell us the story in as much detail as possible. What are we listening for? Missing steps. A few examples might be instructive.

PARENT: Plan B isn't working.

THERAPIST: No? Tell me.

PARENT: Well, on Tuesday I told Curt that I wanted to make sure he got his homework done before his baseball game and asked him how we could work that out.

THERAPIST: So your concern was that he wouldn't get his homework done before his baseball game?

PARENT: Right. I know that if he doesn't do his homework before his baseball game it's not going to get done because by the time we get home from his baseball game he's too tired.

THERAPIST: I see. And what was it that you were trying to work out?

PARENT: What were we trying to work out? How we were going to get his homework done before his baseball game.

THERAPIST: What was *his* concern?

PARENT: His concern?

THERAPIST: Yes, at the moment I'm only hearing *your* concern, which is that you were worried that he wouldn't get his homework done, and your *solution*, which is that he do his homework before his baseball game. What was *his* concern?

PARENT: I didn't know he had a concern.

THERAPIST: Well, at least in your telling of the story, that may be because you skipped the first step of Plan B . . . empathy.

PARENT: I knew I was doing something wrong!

THERAPIST: No one does very well at this in the beginning. What happened when you told him your concern and invited him to solve the problem with you?

PARENT: He started screaming at me.

THERAPIST: Sounds like he must have had a concern. The problem is, when you skip the empathy part and jump right to your concern, he thinks you're using Plan A.

PARENT: Oh my . . . so what should I have said?

THERAPIST: Well, do you have any ideas about what concern he might have had about doing his homework before his baseball game? Has this come up before?

PARENT: Oh, it comes up all the time. He says he needs a break before he does his homework.

THERAPIST: Why does he need a break?

PARENT: Well, he's been in school all day . . . this is what *he* says . . . to tell you the truth, I don't know how hard he's actually working in school . . . anyways, he always seems to have enough energy for baseball . . .

THERAPIST: But I suppose it makes some sense that if he's been in school for 6 hours he might need a break before he jumps right into homework. Sounds like a valid concern to me, if that's what his concern actually is.

PARENT: I suppose so.

THERAPIST: So let's think of what empathy might have sounded like. What could you have said if you wanted to start Plan B off with empathy?

PARENT: Um . . . you mean something like "You're tired?"

THERAPIST: That's a start. Then you can follow the empathy with your concern. See, then you've actually got a problem to solve. Remember, you don't have a problem to solve until you've got two concerns on the table.

PARENT: Ugh! This is hard!

THERAPIST: It takes a little getting used to. But we don't want you to miss out on the good stuff empathy brings to the mix . . . it keeps him calm and it gets his concern on the table.

PARENT: So how would we have solved the problem?

THERAPIST: I don't know how you would have ultimately solved the problem . . . that's between you guys . . . but I'm betting there are lots of possibilities. Of course, we don't uncover those possibilities unless we're using Plan B. Should we invite him into the office and see if he has any ideas for how you guys could solve that problem once and for all?

The above dialogue depicts a classic case of skipping empathy and trying to solve a problem with only the adult concern on the table. We find that some adults skip the empathy step because they have habitually done so and simply need to add an extra step to their repertoire. But, as we mentioned above, other adults . . . sadly, quite a few . . . don't know how to empathize and don't have the skills to formulate the child's concern. We think that's because Plan

A—which has been the conventional approach to childrearing—doesn't train empathy. We find that we often have to train empathy skills to adults and, because it's simpler, we start by training the form of empathy—reflective listening—that would be more commonly found if one were using Emergency Plan B. Here's how it might sound:

THERAPIST: Mr. Johnson, in many of the stories you're telling me about how you've tried to use Plan B, I'm noticing that the empathy step is missing.

MR. JOHNSON: Yes, I'm still trying to get good at that part.

THERAPIST: What do you say we practice a little?

MR. JOHNSON: Practice? You mean, now?

THERAPIST: Sure . . . should we give it a try?

MR. JOHNSON: Well, OK.

THERAPIST: I'm going to say something, and I'd like you to say it right after me.

MR. JOHNSON: OK.

THERAPIST: So I'll say something and you say it right after.

MR. JOHNSON: I'm with ya.

THERAPIST: I want pizza.

MR. JOHNSON: OK.

THERAPIST: Now, you say it.

MR. JOHNSON: I want pizza.

THERAPIST: Say it like you would if you wanted to empathize with me.

MR. JOHNSON: Oh, I gotcha. Uhm, you can have it later.

THERAPIST: Well, now, "you can have it later" is actually a solution, but it's not empathy.

MR. JOHNSON: You sure I'm gonna be able to do this?

THERAPIST: You'll be great. But let's try again. I said "I want pizza." So, if you were just trying to summarize what I just said, you'd say, "You want pizza." Yes?

MR. JOHNSON: (*laughing*) Oh, for goodness sakes, I can do that!

THERAPIST: (*laughing*) Shall we try another?

MR. JOHNSON: Sure thing.

THERAPIST: I want ice cream before dinner.

MR. JOHNSON: You want ice cream before dinner. But you can't . . .

THERAPIST: Hold on! Not so fast! We're just practicing the first step! You did a great job of empathizing. You were about to slide into Plan A, but let's make sure we've got the first step mastered. One more?

MR. JOHNSON: Sure.

THERAPIST: I want to stay up late tonight.

MR. JOHNSON: You want to say up late tonight.

THERAPIST: Outstanding. Now, one last problem.

MR. JOHNSON: Uh-oh. What's the matter?

THERAPIST: Well, we don't quite have any concerns on the table yet.

MR. JOHNSON: We don't?

THERAPIST: No, believe it or not, you'd want to follow your initial empathy with something like "What's up?" so as to clarify the concerns that might have prompted a desire for pizza or ice cream before dinner or to stay up late at night.

MR. JOHNSON: OK, let's try it.

THERAPIST: I want pizza.

MR. JOHNSON: You want pizza. What's up?

THERAPIST: Fabulous. You are now officially an empathizer.

MR. JOHNSON: Do I get a certificate?

THERAPIST: Sorry, no certificates. Of course, the true test is for you to practice this at home, and that's harder.

There are some serious problems that can challenge even the most empathic of humans. It's no easy task to be empathic with an adolescent who, for example, is practicing unsafe sex, using illicit substances, affiliating with deviant peers, lying, or stealing. But it can be done. And if the adult wants to actually talk to the adolescent about these issues, Proactive Plan B is the only way to get it done. With Emergency B, there's added heat. Plan A slams the door shut. With Plan C, the conversation never takes place.

PARENT: I'm pretty certain that Christine is having sex with her boyfriend.

THERAPIST: I suspect you may be right. How do you feel about that?

PARENT: I'm not happy about it. I mean, she's only 15. But there's not a whole lot I can do about it. What am I going to do, lock her in her room?

THERAPIST: I don't suppose that's an option. But why don't you think you can talk to her about it?

PARENT: She won't talk about it!

THERAPIST: What plan have you used in approaching her about the topic?

PARENT: What plan? (*smiling*) That's a good question. I've probably been using Plan A, now that I think of it.

THERAPIST: Plan A doesn't do a very good job of getting the conversation going. And she's still having sex with her boyfriend.

PARENT: I wouldn't have the slightest idea of how to talk about this using Plan B.

THERAPIST: Well, let's think about it. Plan B starts with empathy. How would we get her concern, or at least her point of view, on the table?

PARENT: I really don't know what her concern or point of view is.

THERAPIST: That's OK . . . that's what we're interested in finding out. So maybe we should start with something more general, like "I know you've been seeing Kenny for a long time now . . . I guess you guys are getting pretty close."

PARENT: Sounds good to me.

THERAPIST: Yes, but of course we need to go a little further. If she confirms that she and Kenny are getting pretty close, you could continue with something like, "I know that when people get very close, sometimes they want to show each other how they feel, or sometimes there's pressure to do things that one of them may not be completely comfortable doing." I think that's open-ended enough so that she won't get completely defensive and might actually tell us her point of view. What do you think?

PARENT: I think I'm OK.

THERAPIST: Now, what's your concern?

PARENT: She's too young . . . and I'm afraid she'll get pregnant.

THERAPIST: The pregnant part is pretty specific . . . but I think you'll have to be more specific about her being too young. What is it about her having sex with her boyfriend at the age of 15 that concerns you?

PARENT: Come on! Would you want your daughter having sex with her boyfriend when she's 15?!

THERAPIST: I'm not thrilled at the prospect.

PARENT: See?

THERAPIST: I'm not saying you don't have a valid concern. I'm saying that to have this conversation with Christine you'll have to be more specific about what your concerns are.

PARENT: I don't know if she can handle all the feelings that go along with having sex with someone. And I'm concerned about her reputation.

THERAPIST: I think we've got your concerns identified. I think your concerns are wonderful. By the way, I suspect she has legitimate concerns, too. I might alter the invitation a little bit . . . maybe something like, "Can we talk about this?"

PARENT: Yes . . . I think that's a good idea.

THERAPIST: So I think you're ready to take a stab at this conversation. What do you think . . . would it be better for you two to have this conversation at home or in my office?

PARENT: I think I'd like to try it at home. I don't know if she wants to talk about it in here. What do you think?

THERAPIST: I think that's fine. Now, do you think this is a one-time conversation? I mean, is this something that's going to get resolved in 5 minutes?

PARENT: I doubt it.

THERAPIST: I agree . . . and if the first conversation doesn't go so well, make sure you at least set the stage for the topic to come up again.

Naturally, if an adult is having difficulty being highly specific about his or her concerns in the "define the problem" step of Plan B, the Plan B discussion will veer off course. In such instances, the role of the therapist is to help the adult identify and articulate his or her concerns and to remind the adult of the difference between a concern and a solution. The following is an example of how such a discussion might sound; in this instance, the child is also in the room and there are 5 minutes left in the session:

CHILD: I wanna call my dad.

MOTHER: No.

THERAPIST: (to mother) That's Plan A, you know.

MOTHER: Plan A?

THERAPIST: (to mother) Yes . . . he said he wanted to call his dad and you said no. That's Plan A.

MOTHER: But I don't want him to call his father.

THERAPIST: (*to mother*) I gathered. But I don't know *why* you don't want him to call his father. In other words, I know your *solution* but I don't know what your *concern* is.

MOTHER: My concern? You mean, why don't I want him to call his father? Hmm . . . now that's an interesting question . . . Um (*laughing*) . . . my concern . . . I think it's because I don't want him to interrupt us.

THERAPIST: That's a wonderful concern . . . now we can do Plan B. (*turning to child*) You want to call your dad . . . your mom wants to make sure you don't interrupt us. Can you think of how we can work that out?

CHILD: How 'bout I talk softly.

THERAPIST: (*to mother*) Do you have any objections to his calling his father right now besides that he might interrupt us?

MOTHER: I don't think so.

THERAPIST: Does his solution . . . talking softly . . . work for you?

MOTHER: (*hesitatingly*) Yes . . . I think it does.

THERAPIST: (*to child*) Does it work for you?

CHILD: Yup.

THERAPIST: (*to child*) You sure you're going to be able to talk softly? I don't want you agreeing to something you can't do.

CHILD: I can talk softly. Does that mean I can call my dad?

THERAPIST: (*to child*) Yes, I think it does.

MOTHER: (*whispering to therapist*) Did we just give in?

THERAPIST: (*to mother*) I don't think so. But let's think about it. Your concern was that he would interrupt us and we addressed that concern. How did we give in?

MOTHER: Well, he still got to call his father.

THERAPIST: Yes, he got to call his father because we were able to identify your concern and come up with a solution that addressed that concern. That's not giving in . . . that's *problem solving*. If you head straight for Plan A with your concern, the problem won't get solved . . . it'll just get worse.

MOTHER: So I need to figure out what my concern is?

THERAPIST: That's right . . . if you don't lay your concern on the table, he won't be able to take your needs into account.

MOTHER: He doesn't take my needs into account anyway.

THERAPIST: Sounds like you both need some practice.

MOTHER: This is hard.

THERAPIST: Yes, it is. Many parents don't need to think about why they said no because they've got children who can handle no. But you have a child who doesn't handle no very well . . . for all the reasons we've discussed already . . . so we have to be more careful with the word "no" in his case and set the stage for you guys to practice working on the problem together. If you don't get two concerns on the table, no one gets any practice.

Finally, as we mentioned briefly above, it is quite common for adults to do a fine job with the empathy and problem definition steps and then jump straight into the Plan A frying pan by skipping the invitation. In such instances, the therapist's role is to notice that a Plan B step is missing, provide feedback along these lines, and provide opportunities for practice:

PARENT: We had a big blowout this week.

THERAPIST: I'm sorry. Over what?

PARENT: Gymnastics. And I was doing Plan B!

THERAPIST: What's the problem with gymnastics?

PARENT: He doesn't want to go.

THERAPIST: So tell me what happened.

PARENT: I told him that I understood he didn't want to go to gymnastics but that we had already paid for the class so he needed to go.

THERAPIST: So let me make sure I've got this straight. He doesn't want to go to gymnastics . . . do you know why?

PARENT: He says it's boring.

THERAPIST: And you've let him know that you're aware of the fact that he thinks gym is boring?

PARENT: Oh, absolutely.

THERAPIST: Who wants him to go to gymnastics?

PARENT: Me! He's always quitting everything. I can't tell you how much money we've wasted on things he's started and then decided to quit.

THERAPIST: OK, so I think we've figured out what the two concerns are . . . he thinks gym is boring and you're not so thrilled about him quitting or about losing money. Yes?

PARENT: Yes.

THERAPIST: I take it this has come up before.

PARENT: All the time.

THERAPIST: So this conversation you had with him is taking place just before you're about to leave for gym?

PARENT: Right.

THERAPIST: I do want to hear what happened next, but I must say there are probably more opportune moments to have this discussion besides just as you're about to leave for gym.

PARENT: Like when?

THERAPIST: Like any time *besides* when you're about to leave for gym. At bedtime the night before, over the weekend, when you're in the car together . . . you know, some time when you guys aren't so heated up.

PARENT: I see your point.

THERAPIST: But let's get back to the problem. He doesn't want to go to gym because it's boring and you don't want him to quit because you've paid good money. I think we've got the problem defined, yes?

PARENT: Yes.

THERAPIST: So, what solutions did he come up with to solve the problem?

PARENT: Well, his solution was that he shouldn't go.

THERAPIST: That was his solution to *his* concern. What was his solution once you got *both* concerns on the table?

PARENT: I don't know.

THERAPIST: Did he have any ideas?

PARENT: I don't know . . . I think I didn't ask.

THERAPIST: Oh . . . now I understand . . . he never got invited to solve the problem with you.

PARENT: Right. I guess I pretty much told him what the solution was, so he never got a chance to help out with the solution.

THERAPIST: So the third step—the invitation—was missing.

PARENT: Right.

THERAPIST: How did he respond to your solution . . . you know, that he go to the gym anyway?

PARENT: He went nuts.

THERAPIST: That's because your solution didn't take his concern into account, which means it wasn't mutually acceptable.

PARENT: So remind me what should I have said again.

THERAPIST: Well, the invitation usually sounds something like "Let's think of how we can work that out" or "Let's think of how we can solve that problem." The word "let's" lets him know that solving the problem is something you're doing *with* him, not *to* him.

PARENT: I don't think he's going to have any ideas.

THERAPIST: You might be right . . . on the other hand, he might surprise you. If you're right, and he truly has no ideas for how to solve the problem, it may be because he's become accustomed to you solving the problem for him. So giving him practice at coming up with solutions is all the more important. If he can't come up with any solutions, then it's fine for you to kick in with some tentative ideas. Remember, the ideas that will work are the ones that are mutually acceptable . . . that take your concerns *and* his concerns into account.

PARENT: I do like to solve problems for him, don't I?

THERAPIST: It's certainly starting to look that way. But let's practice . . . let's get him in here and see whether he's as devoid of solutions as we might think.

We often tell adults that an important assessment opportunity occurs right after a child has been invited to help solve a problem: *Does the child have any skills at generating alternative solutions? Is he able to generate solutions that take both concerns into account?* As suggested elsewhere, sometimes the reason a child is not very good at solving problems is because adults don't provide opportunities for doing so. In other instances, however, it's because specific skill deficits are interfering. If a child has difficulty generating solutions and taking others' concerns into account, the role of the surrogate frontal lobe is clear: Help the child learn to generate alternative solutions to problems and take others' concerns into account. We have more to say about this topic in Chapter 6.

Interestingly, one reason adults fail to invite a child to assist in solving a problem is that they (the adults) do not have any ideas themselves. As one mother we worked with explained, "I think the reason I end up using Plan A sometimes is because I can't think of anything either! I can't use Plan B if I don't know how to solve the problem in the first place, right?" Actually, not right. We explained to this mom that she actually doesn't have to have a great solution at the ready to invite the child to collaboratively solve the problem. The job of the surrogate frontal lobe is not to solve the problem for the child but to help the child participate in solving it together.

Q & A

I've seen instances in which the child or adolescent grew tired of the reflective listening form of empathy. What then?

Well, reflective listening is the form of empathy associated with *Emergency* Plan B. So one reason the kid tires of reflective listening is that the adults are overusing *Emergency* Plan B and underutilizing *Proactive* Plan B. But adolescents in particular tend to react poorly when they feel like their adult interaction partner is acting alike a mental health professional, and reflective listening can make some kids feel that way. In these instances, reflective listening can be replaced with a simple "I hear ya."

What if the first solution doesn't work? What if the child won't do his part of the solution?

It's extremely common in the human experience that the first solution to a problem fails to solve the problem durably. In fact, most good solutions are the by-product of preceding solutions that didn't completely get the job done. Solutions that don't stand the test of time should inform modifications to the original solution. So if a child (or adult) isn't willing or able to carry out his or her part of a solution, it's usually a sign that the solution wasn't feasible, doable, or mutually satisfactory, and it's back to the Plan B drawing board. More on this topic in Chapter 6.

There are some issues mentioned only briefly above that I'd like some additional guidance on, especially lying and stealing. How would these issues be handled with Plan B?

The steps are the same. Just remember, some difficult issues require more than one Plan B conversation. Sometimes the solution that ends up solving the problem durably isn't found until after a few solutions to the problem have been tried. Here's how a Proactive Plan B conversation might sound on the lying issue:

ADULT: (*empathy*) I've noticed that sometimes it's hard for you to tell me the truth about some things.

CHILD: Like what?

ADULT: Well, the other day I asked you if your homework was done and you told me it was. So I let you keep playing your video game. But I got a note from Mrs. Nixon today that your homework actually wasn't done.

CHILD: She's lying!

ADULT: (*empathy*) She could be lying, I guess. But I've noticed that you were having trouble telling the truth about some other things that had nothing to do with Mrs. Nixon.

CHILD: What else?

ADULT: Um, when I called home from my meeting last week I asked you if you had mowed the lawn yet and you told me you did. And then I got home and the lawn wasn't mowed. Remember?

CHILD: Well, I meant to mow the lawn before you got home, but I didn't get to it.

ADULT: (*empathy, then defining the problem*) I understand how that could happen. The thing is, when you lie to me about those things it makes me feel like I can't trust you on other things.

CHILD: OK, I won't lie anymore!

ADULT: (*clarifying the problem*) Um, that would be wonderful. But I think I'd feel a little more confident about that if I understood why you were having trouble telling me the truth in the first place.

CHILD: I don't want you to get mad at me. I don't want you to scream at me.

ADULT: (*empathy*) Ah, you don't want me to get mad and scream at you. I can understand that. I guess I can get pretty mad about things, can't I?

CHILD: Yup.

ADULT: (*redefining the problem, then invitation*) OK, so you sometimes have trouble telling me the truth because you don't want me to get mad and scream at you. And I want to feel like I can trust you to tell the truth. Let's think about what we can do about that. You have any ideas?

CHILD: You could promise not to scream at me.

ADULT: I could promise that. Except I don't know if I can keep that promise all the time. I might slip sometimes. I can promise to try very hard not to scream at you. Have you noticed I've been screaming a lot less lately?

CHILD: Yes. I could promise to try very hard not to lie to you.

ADULT: So we both have something to work on, don't we?

CHILD: Yup.

ADULT: What should we do if I slip up and start screaming?

CHILD: I could remind you of your promise.

ADULT: That would be very helpful. What should I do if you slip up and tell me a lie?

CHILD: You could remind me of my promise.

ADULT: I think we've got a plan. Let's see how it works. If it doesn't work too well we'll talk again and see if we can figure out what to do instead.

CHILD: OK.

ADULT: Great. Now, how about we talk about the homework?

Shouldn't safety be handled with Plan A?

In previous variants of the CPS model, safety was handled exclusively with Plan A. But then we noticed that a lot of families who were doing a good job of executing Plan B on nonsafety issues were still experiencing many explosive episodes over the safety issues they had handled with Plan A. In other words, the problems that were causing safety issues weren't being resolved because these problems were being handled with Plan A. So we have a new mantra: the first time adults notice that a child is exhibiting an urgent unsafe behavior—placing a hand on a hot stove, walking in front of a moving car in parking lot, and so on—handle it with Plan A because there's no time to do Plan B. But if, after numerous repetitions of Plan A on these or similar safety problems, the child is still exhibiting the unsafe behavior, you're probably going to have to identify pathways and triggers and get the job done through Proactive Plan B.

This brings up an interesting point. A lot of parents and teachers tell me they don't have time to do Plan B. What's your response?

Our response is that they don't have time *not* to do Plan B. As we've noted in previous chapters, explosive episodes always take more time than Plan B. Unsolved problems always take more time than solved problems. Let us paraphrase: continuing to implement an intervention that isn't fixing the problem is very time- and labor-intensive and simply heightens frustration in child and adults. Once a problem is durably solved, it doesn't require much time at all anymore.

How is "working it out" different from "compromising" or "negotiating"?

There is a lot of overlap between the terms. But many adults think "compromising" means always "meeting halfway" on a solution, and there are many mutually satisfactory solutions that do not involve meeting half-way. And we've found that many adults who were unwilling to "negotiate" with a child—conventional wisdom has convinced them that it was a bad idea to do so—were perfectly willing to work toward a mutually satisfactory solution that addressed the concerns of adult and child. So we tend to avoid the terms "compromising" and "negotiating."

What about nagging? What plan is that?

Well, nagging does present the child with an expectation, so it wouldn't be Plan C. And nagging certainly isn't an attempt to solve a problem collaboratively, so it certainly wouldn't be Plan B. Which leaves us with only one remaining option. Plan A. Annoying, apprehensive Plan A, perhaps, but definitely Plan A.

How do you introduce the three plans to adult caretakers? Exactly what words do you use?

We typically introduce the plans in much same way that they have been described in this chapter. That being said, clinicians often like to hear exactly what it sounds like in a session. Let's listen in toward the end of a typical first session:

THERAPIST: Well, now that we have some sense of the lagging skills that are setting the stage for Jen to have such a hard time handling frustration, we need to give some thought to how we're going to teach those skills and to how to solve problems in a way that doesn't cause explosions.

MRS. J: Good.

THERAPIST: There's basically three ways in which adults pursue expectations and solve problems with children. We call those three options Plan A, Plan B, and Plan C. Whenever you're solving a problem, or handling a disagreement, or pursuing an expectation with Jen, you're probably using one of those plans.

MRS. J: OK.

THERAPIST: Plan A is, quite simply, when you impose your will in response to a problem or unmet expectation. Among most adults, that's a very popular option. Plan C is when you drop the expectation completely. And Plan B is when you work things out with her in a way that makes you both happy.

MR. J: So Plan C is where you decide to give in because it's not worth a big blow-out? We do a lot of that.

THERAPIST: Well, Plan C isn't quite the same thing as giving in. The definition of "giving in" is when you start with Plan A and end up using Plan C because Jen made your life miserable. But when you start with Plan C, you're making the conscious decision not to pursue a given expectation, either because you've decided it's not as high a priority as some of your other concerns, because you've concluded that the expectation involves skills that Jen doesn't yet possess, or because you've decided it's going to be necessary to drop some expectations, at least temporarily, to reduce the global level of tension in your household.

MR. J: I got it. This is like picking your battles. We do a lot of that with Jen already.

THERAPIST: I wouldn't exactly call this picking your battles. In our experience, picking battles is just choosing between Plan A and Plan C. Once I explain what Plan B looks like, you'll see that this approach really has very little to do with picking battles.

MR. J: I'm open to all this, but I honestly think we do a lot of each plan already. Lord knows we use plenty of Plan A! And I think we've also lowered our expectations quite a bit. And we talk to Jen all the time.

THERAPIST: Well, Plan B is a bit more involved than simply talking. In fact, there are some specific steps involved in doing Plan B. We'll get to the steps in a second, but I should also tell you that one of our goals is for you to be doing a lot less of Plan A.

MR. J: Less Plan A?

THERAPIST: Yes. I'm betting that if we rewound the tape on most of the explosions that occur in your household, what we'd find is an adult using Plan A. An important part of reducing explosions in your household is having you use Plan A a lot less. Instead, we want to proceed in a way that helps you pursue expectations without causing explosions, while simultaneously teaching Jen the thinking skills she needs to handle frustration better than she does now. When you're using Plan A, only one of those goals—pursuing expectations—is being achieved. Again, you're not *reducing* explosions by imposing your will, you're *causing* them. And you don't teach Jen how to be less black-and-white or how to express her needs more adaptively by imposing your will. So Plan A isn't going to be a big part of your future.

MR. J: So how do we get her to do what she needs to do?

THERAPIST: That would be Plan B. But let me tell you about Plan C first. With Plan C, you're dropping an expectation, thereby preventing an explosion. But with Plan C, you're not pursuing an expectation and you're not teaching any new skills. So Plan C—which will be very useful to us early on, as we try to reduce the global level of tension and frustration in your family—isn't the plan that will be most important over time.

MR. J: Which leads us to Plan B.

THERAPIST: Correct. Plan B is a way to pursue expectations without causing an explosion, and simultaneously teach skills that will help her handle frustration more adaptively moving forward.

MRS. J: So all this time we've been using Plan A to try to correct the problem, and it really hasn't been correcting the problem at all. I feel terrible.

THERAPIST: If it makes you feel any better, most adults are taught to think that Plan A is the best way to get the job done. And a lot of parents can get by with Plan A. But you can't. Jen is going to require a specialized approach to parenting. And that's Plan B.

MRS. J: OK. So how do we do Plan B?

THERAPIST: Well, first I should tell you that there are two forms of Plan B: Emergency B and Proactive B. Emergency B is where you're waiting until you're right in the middle of a problem or disagreement to use Plan B, and it's not ideal timing because people are starting to get heated up already. Proactive B is where you're trying to solve a predictable problem before it comes up again. In most families, the same problems cause explosions day after day and week after week. We call these "problems that have yet to be solved," because we know if they'd been solved already people wouldn't still be exploding because of them.

MRS. J: Makes sense.

THERAPIST: One of my jobs is to help you guys identify the problems that are predictably causing explosions in your household and then to help you use Proactive Plan B to solve them once and for all. Now, there are three steps involved in doing Plan B. The first step is empathy. There are a few reasons Plan B starts with empathy. First, empathy tends to keep people calm. People—not just kids—tend to stay calm when they're feeling heard and understood. Second, empathy ensures that Jen's concern is on the table. We won't be able to solve the problem unless Jen's concern is on the table. It's only in this first step that Proactive B and Emergency B differ. With Emergency B, you're simply trying to reflect back to Jen whatever she just said. Let's take the example you gave earlier when Jen wanted to go to the movies with her friends on Sunday night. If she had said, "I want to go to the movies," you could have said, "You want to go to the movies," and that would have been a fine example of empathy. Proactive B always starts with, "I've noticed that. . . . " So if Jen going to the movies with her friends on Sunday nights was routinely causing a problem, and you wanted to handle the problem proactively, then empathy would be something like, "I've noticed that you always want to go to the movies with your friends on Sunday nights." Still with me?

MRS. J: I think so.

THERAPIST: Now, I should point out . . . and this is where things might get a bit confusing . . . that we haven't yet established why it's so important to Jen that she go to the movies with her friends on Sunday nights, so we don't really have her concern on the table yet. Any theories?

MRS. J: She'd say that she only gets to spend time with these friends on the weekends, which is true.

THERAPIST: Excellent. If we didn't know that . . . or if we weren't sure what her concern was . . . then after our initial stab at empathy—"I've noticed that you always want to go to the movies with your friends on Sunday nights"—we might add a question like, "What's up?" If she responds the way you think she will, then we can follow with a more refined form of empathy, something like "Ah, you want to go to the movies with them on Sunday nights because you don't get to spend much time with them except on weekends." Now we've empathized and we're ready to move to the second step of Plan B. We call it the Define the Problem step. This is when you put your concern on the table. What's your concern about her going to the movies with her friends on Sunday nights?

MR. J: Our concern is that she gets very little homework done over the weekend and so she doesn't usually get to it until Sunday night. If she's at the movies the homework won't get done.

THERAPIST: Sounds like a valid concern. How would you say it to her?

MR. J: I'd say you can't go to the movies with your friends because you have to get your homework done.

THERAPIST: Well, you just put your solution on the table, but not your concern. This is the hardest part of doing Plan B. Your solution is that she not go to the movies . . . but your concern is that her homework won't get done.

MR. J: OK, I'm with you. This *is* hard.

THERAPIST: Getting two solutions on the table instead of two concerns is probably the most common stumbling block for people new to Plan B.

MR. J: I'd say that's one we're going to need some practice on.

THERAPIST: See, the reason we call the second step Define the Problem is that we define a problem simply as two concerns that have yet to be reconciled. Her concern and your concern. But if we don't have two concerns on the table, we won't know what problem we're trying to solve.

MR. J: Hold on, though. The second I tell her my concern she's going to get all upset because she knows we're going to say no to the movies.

THERAPIST: But with Plan B, you aren't going to say no. You aren't going to say yes, either. Plan B is neither agreeing nor disagreeing, neither yes nor no. With Plan B you're going to try to find a solution to the problem that works for everyone.

MR. J: OK, but she doesn't know that so she'll probably start to get all upset as soon as we bring up our concern.

THERAPIST: Well, sometimes we add a little reassurance to the empathy to keep her calm.

MR. J: Reassurance?

THERAPIST: Yes, reassurance that you're not using Plan A. Of course, she doesn't know what Plan A is, so you can't say, "I'm not using Plan A." But you can say something like, "I'm not saying you can't go to the movies." You then re-empathize with her concern and remind her of yours. So far so good?

MRS. J: I think so.

THERAPIST: Don't worry, you're going to have lots of opportunities to practice! The third step of Plan B is called the Invitation. That's when you're inviting Jen to brainstorm solutions with you that will solve the problem.

MR. J: OK. But let's say she says, "How about if I get the homework done before I go to the movies?" Are we supposed to be OK with that?

THERAPIST: That's up to you. Our litmus test for good solutions is that they be realistic, doable, and mutually satisfactory. If a solution isn't realistic or doable then it won't stand the test of time. And if it's not mutually satisfactory, then someone's concern isn't being addressed. Does that solution—her doing her homework before she goes to the movies—work for you? Does it address your concern?

MR. J: Sure . . . if she'll actually do it.

THERAPIST: Do you think she can do it?

MRS. J: I think we'd need to help her plan her weekends a little better.

THERAPIST: Well, it sounds like it could be realistic with a little fine-tuning. Of course, we're missing a very important person here. If we were truly doing collaborative problem solving, we'd need Jen in here with us. But if the solution isn't realistic, doable, and mutually satisfactory, then you're still brainstorming. And she may need a little more reassurance thrown into the process to let her know that you are confident that you guys will be able to come up with a solution that will address her concern.

MR. J: So it's her job to come up with the solutions?

THERAPIST: No, it's everyone's job to come up with solutions. It's good strategy to give her first crack at it, though. Just remember, there's a pretty good chance that her initial solutions won't be realistic, doable, or mutually satisfactory.

MR. J: You got that right! Her first solution is going to be whatever works for her!

THERAPIST: But remember that's because Jen is a black-and-white thinker who has difficulty generating solutions to problems that take other's needs into account. All the more reason to do Plan B. She needs the practice. Of course, it could also be the case that she's accustomed to having solutions offered to her that only work for the person offering the solution.

MRS. J: Ah, yes . . . a very distinct possibility. So what if we agree on something and she doesn't follow through on her end?

THERAPIST: Then you're back to Plan B to figure out why and come up with something more realistic, doable, or mutually satisfactory. I should warn you that most initial solutions don't durably solve most problems for most people. Most good, durable solutions come after solutions that didn't quite get the job done.

MR. J: This is going to take some time!

THERAPIST: It is, but it's not going to take any more time than you've been spending fighting with each other. And I'm optimistic you'll have a lot more to show for your time and hard work because you'll be solving problems in a way that ensures they aren't problems anymore. Nothing is harder than problems that never get solved.

MR. J: When do we use Emergency Plan B?

THERAPIST: When something pops up unexpectedly. Otherwise, you're trying to solve problems proactively, way before they pop up.

MRS. J: Well, we can try.

THERAPIST: Just remember, it takes most folks a while to get the hang of it. So what we'll do in future sessions is try to fine-tune your attempts to use Plan B and try to tackle one problem at a time.

Chapter 5

Beyond the Basics

You now know that helping adults and children master Plan B is crucial to the successful implementation of the CPS model. Plan B is not a behavior management technique; rather, it is a framework through which adults and children communicate, problem-solve, and resolve conflict more adaptively, thereby setting in motion fundamental and durable changes in adult–child interactions. By the way, Plan B is also a means of *assessment*—as families begin to attempt to solve problems collaboratively, factors interfering with implementation of Plan B often become readily apparent. For example, certain skills are necessary for adults and kids to participate in Plan B discussions: identifying and articulating each other's concerns; taking another's concerns into account in generating alternative solutions; and anticipating the likely outcomes of solutions. Plan B discussions provide rich and directly observable information about each participant's skills in these (and other) domains, and it is the therapist's role to identify lagging skills and set the stage for their remediation (a topic we've saved for Chapter 6). For Plan B discussions to take place in the therapist's office—and for participants to be receptive to feedback on factors that may be impeding these discussions—the therapist must also facilitate a *therapeutic process* through which Plan B can be modeled, practiced, fine-tuned, embraced, and (ultimately) implemented independently. To achieve this goal, the therapist must establish alliances with each participant; maintain a (largely) neutral stance on the issues and problems being discussed; determine whether and when family members are able to converse directly with each other and actively prevent discussions from spinning out of control; be on the lookout for conflicting guidance that may be hindering participants' full investment in implementation; help participants stay on track in their discussions and in their expectations about the anticipated rate of progress; and be attentive to and prepared to address family systems issues that may be hampering collaborative problem solving. These roles are the focus of this chapter.

ESTABLISHING ALLIANCES

The single greatest predictor of therapeutic change—and this is true of all forms of psychotherapy—is the degree to which a therapeutic alliance is achieved between clinicians and patients. CPS frequently requires a shift in mind-set and always requires hard work—often, extremely hard work. In implementing CPS, things often get worse before they get better. In fact, psychopathology is likely to be in full bloom the week after adults try to implement Plan B for the first time. The therapist's relationship with the child and adult caretakers is often essential to seeing people through the hard times. Establishing an alliance with those participating in treatment is crucial.

All the usual tools come into play here. In Chapter 2 we suggested that adults don't need large doses of empathy for an alliance to be established, and that the best way for the therapist to communicate empathy is by asking questions that demonstrate an understanding of explosive children and an ability to home in on the factors underlying a given child's difficulties. Nonetheless, additional empathy may be important in a number of areas: how hard it is to ask for help (from a stranger, no less); how difficult, embarrassing, humiliating, isolating, and frustrating it can be to deal with a behaviorally challenging child; how hard it is to admit to feeling overwhelmed and helpless and to air dirty laundry; how (justifiably) skeptical adults can be that anyone will be able to get a handle on a child's difficulties; how hard it can be to feel comfortable and confident in collaboratively solving problems with a child. Of course, adult caretakers not only need to be heard and understood; they also need to feel that the clinician has the capacity to durably relieve their distress.

A similar alliance must also be established with the child. Many children resonate to the idea that the therapist can help the child and his adult caretakers get along better. Of course, some children come into therapy with no prior experience with helping professionals and are therefore fairly clueless about what they've been dragged into. Some of these children simply need to be re-assured that they are not about to be on the receiving end of an injection. The rest are usually initially easily engaged through casual conversation or a game. Others come into therapy with mixed or largely unpleasant prior experiences with helping professionals. These kids will need some reassurance that things may be a little different this time around. In our experience, once the child feels heard, understands that you do not think that he is intentionally behaving poorly, and is clear on the fact that the clinician views his situation as a "family problem" rather than as solely "his problem," he is closer to being on board. As mentioned in Chapter 2, adolescents sometimes require special handling, but in general they are just as receptive to being heard and understood as anyone else. Occasionally, of course, there is the child who is very angry about being brought to therapy and refuses to engage. Empathy is still the name of the game here: "I'm sorry you had to come here when you didn't want to." In the case of one 8-year-old boy who presented as extremely depressed and refused to speak at all, the therapist asked that the boy simply raise his index finger if the therapist made an accurate statement. The therapist then began speaking for the boy.

THERAPIST: I guess you're pretty mad about being here today.

BOY: (*no finger*).

THERAPIST: I think they brought you because they're concerned about how you sometimes lose your temper.

BOY: (*no finger*).

THERAPIST: Hmm . . . maybe they should have brought you here because they're concerned about how *they* sometimes lose *their* tempers.

BOY: (*raised finger*).

THERAPIST: What do they do when they lose their tempers?

BOY: (*no finger*).

THERAPIST: Do they scream at you?

BOY: (*raised finger*).

THERAPIST: I'm sorry about that. Do they hit you?

BOY: With a belt.

THERAPIST: That's not OK, is it?

BOY: No, it isn't.

THERAPIST: Do they both hit you with a belt?

BOY: Mostly my dad.

THERAPIST: Would you like me to help them stop screaming at you and hitting you with the belt?

BOY: (*nodding*).

MAINTAINING NEUTRALITY (MOST OF THE TIME)

Because therapists are trained to be empathic and supportive, there is a temptation, in almost any form of therapy, to ally oneself with the "offended party." Moreover, parents and children often come into therapy with the expectation that the therapist will be the arbiter of right and wrong. It's no accident that people have this mind-set, for (unfortunately) we live in an era where "winning" versus "losing" and rigid definitions of "right" versus "wrong" pervade many issues facing our society. Thus, when working with children and their adult caretakers, the temptation can break in either direction, such that therapists can find themselves agreeing with the child when they feel that the adults are being unreasonable and agreeing with the adults when they feel that the child is being unreasonable.

In the CPS model, there are much more productive ways to insert oneself into a system than by taking sides. Indeed, it is actually counterproductive for the therapist to take sides. In succumbing to temptation, the therapist assumes the role of power broker. This is not an ideal role. If the therapist is busy meting out justice, when precisely do the parties learn to work things out with each other?

Indeed, the CPS model requires *finely honed neutrality* on the part of the therapist. The role of the therapist is to accurately represent both sides and to ensure that both concerns make it into the discussion ("Mr. Jackson, that sounds like a very reasonable concern . . . let's hear what Jimmy's concerns are about this issue now" or "Sam, I think we're pretty clear about your feeling that you'd like your curfew to be later . . . but I'd also like to hear your parents' concerns about that"). *The best protection against taking sides is remaining focused on understanding and clarifying each person's concerns.*

However, empathy can sometimes be misinterpreted as agreeing with the stance someone has taken, so it is crucial for the therapist to stay the course: while the therapist is acknowledging that a given person's concerns are legitimate, he or she is also pointing out that contrasting concerns are legitimate as well and underscoring the fact that *concerns* and *solutions* are completely different animals. The ultimate goal is to help children and adults work toward a mutually satisfactory outcome, and it is the children and adults—not the therapist—who determine what defines "mutually satisfactory." Therapists can draw inspiration along these lines from the words of the famous therapist (and songwriter) Dave Mason: "There ain't no good guys . . . there ain't no bad guys . . . there's only you and me and we just disagree."

Example 1

CHILD: My parents suck.

THERAPIST: I'm sorry to hear that.

CHILD: Well, don't you think they suck?

THERAPIST: I don't live with them . . . but I know *you* sometimes think they suck.

CHILD: They won't let me get an earring.

THERAPIST: Ah, you want an earring. Why won't they let you get one?

CHILD: Because they suck. Don't you think it's OK for kids to have earrings?

THERAPIST: I haven't really given it much thought . . . of course, I'm not your parents.

CHILD: You're on their side, aren't you?

THERAPIST: I'm not on anyone's side. Actually, I think I may be on everyone's side. I understand that you want an earring and I suspect your parents have some concerns about that. What matters is how you're going to work this out with them.

CHILD: They won't work it out!

THERAPIST: I'm surprised . . . you guys have worked out a lot of things in here over the past few months.

CHILD: They won't even talk about it.

THERAPIST: How do you know they won't talk about it?

CHILD: Every time I bring it up they just say no.

THERAPIST: Do you know what their concern is about you getting an earring?

CHILD: No.

THERAPIST: Why don't I check in with them and find out what their concern is and we'll go from there.

Example 2

PARENT: Javier punched a hole in my wall this week. I think he should pay to have it repaired, don't you?

THERAPIST: What happened?

PARENT: We were arguing about something . . . I can't actually remember what. But don't you think he should pay for the damage he caused?

THERAPIST: I don't know. I know it's very upsetting to have a hole punched in your wall.

PARENT: Well, I can't just let it go like nothing happened.

THERAPIST: No, I suppose not. Can you try to remember what happened that ended up with him punching a hole in the wall?

PARENT: I think we were arguing over whether he should be allowed to sleep over at his friend's house Saturday night.

THERAPIST: You didn't want him to?

PARENT: No, because I didn't know if the kid's parents would be home to supervise. Don't you agree that I shouldn't let him sleep at some kid's house if I don't know if the parents are going to be home?

THERAPIST: What's your concern about that?

PARENT: That he won't be supervised. You never know what kids are going to do if they're unsupervised late at night.

THERAPIST: Sounds like a valid concern to me. So you wanted to make sure the parents were going to be home. Did Javier have a problem with that?

PARENT: No . . . I mean, I don't know.

THERAPIST: You don't know?

PARENT: Well . . . we didn't really talk about that.

THERAPIST: I don't understand.

PARENT: He told me he wanted to sleep over his friend's house. So I told him he couldn't sleep over unless I was sure the parents were home. So then he calls me a name . . . I told him he can't sleep at his friend's house if he's going to call me names . . . he punches a hole in my wall. But all I'm asking is, don't you think he should pay for me to have the hole repaired?

THERAPIST: Well, how the hole gets repaired is certainly something we should talk about. But you realize you were doing Plan A, yes?

PARENT: What, you think I should let him call me names?

THERAPIST: Actually, you were doing Plan A before he called you a name.

PARENT: When?

THERAPIST: When you told him he couldn't sleep at his friend's unless you were sure the parents were going to be home.

PARENT: So I should have let him sleep over even if I wasn't sure the parents were going to be home?

THERAPIST: Well, that would be Plan C. What I'm driving at is that Javier's concern never made it onto the table and he was never invited to solve the problem with you.

PARENT: But I didn't want him sleeping at his friend's house unless the parents were home.

THERAPIST: I know, that was *your* concern. It's just that, if you were trying to do Plan B, *his* concern and the invitation were missing. I think that may be why you have a hole in your wall.

PARENT: So you're saying he shouldn't pay for the hole?

THERAPIST: The hole needs to be discussed . . . but what I am saying is that if the sleepover issue had been handled with Plan B we probably wouldn't be talking about who's paying for the hole right now.

PARENT: OK, so I should've been doing Plan B. Who pays for the hole?

THERAPIST: Well, let's talk about that with Javier . . . but I want to make sure we also discuss the issue that put the hole in the wall in the first place, because it's going to come up again.

Having now established the importance of neutrality, you may have noticed that there are some things about which the CPS clinician is explicitly *non*neutral. As you know, this is certainly the case when explanations for a child's explosive behavior are being discussed, but also when it comes to pointing out that the same adult concern can be addressed via Plan B instead of Plan A; that a child is being over- or undermedicated; that a child might require pharmacotherapy to benefit maximally from psychosocial treatment; that a child is, at least for the time being, so volatile and unstable that Plan C is going to be the primary option until he is more available to participate in and benefit from Plan B. In other words, there are times when a therapist cannot be a Plan B role model, as in the following dialogue:

FATHER: We had a horrible week.

MOTHER: Yes.

THERAPIST: What's going on?

MOTHER: Well, he stopped taking his meds 2 weeks ago . . . he'd only been on the Lexapro 2 weeks before he stopped taking it . . . and we weren't sure if it was working . . . but now, seeing him off it again, we're sure it was working.

THERAPIST: What's he been like?

FATHER: Mean . . . just mean.

THERAPIST: Mean like grouchy, grumpy, irritable?

FATHER: That's putting it mildly. Plus he had three panic attacks this weekend . . . we came very close to putting him in the hospital. We had to threaten to put him in the hospital to get him to start taking his meds again.

THERAPIST: Panic attacks? What did those look like?

FATHER: Completely out of control . . . breathing heavy . . . sweaty palms . . . talking to himself . . .

MOTHER: They weren't panic attacks.

FATHER: They *were* panic attacks . . . I think I know what a panic attack looks like . . .

THERAPIST: What was Ben having panic attacks about . . . anything in particular?

FATHER: Uh . . . no, not really.

MOTHER: Uh . . . *yes*, really.

THERAPIST: Mrs. R, what was going on before Ben had the panic attacks?

MOTHER: His father was yelling at him to go clean his room.

FATHER: Well, his room was dirty. Look, someone's gotta teach this kid how to live with other people.

THERAPIST: (*to father*) So the panic attacks came right after you did Plan A?

FATHER: What am I supposed to do, just sit there while he doesn't listen to anything we say?

MOTHER: To be fair, once Ben stopped taking the meds, he also stopped participating in Plan B. . . . I mean, he just wouldn't talk to us.

THERAPIST: Well, unless I'm missing something, I'm rather doubtful that Ben was having panic attacks. But it does sound to me like we're back to where we were before Ben started taking the meds. The reason we had him start on the Lexapro was because we thought his level of irritability was just so intense that there wasn't much chance he was going to be able to tolerate any kind of discussion about anything. But now he's taking it again?

MOTHER: Yes, for the past 3 days.

THERAPIST: I think we need to get back to the mentality we were in before he started taking the Lexapro. Four weeks ago, we were mostly doing Plan C and hoping that when the meds kicked in Ben would be able to begin participating in Plan B. When he was taking the meds, was there any indication that Plan B was more possible?

FATHER: No.

MOTHER: Not no . . . yes . . . with those of us who were actually trying to do Plan B with him.

THERAPIST: Mr. R, I'm concerned that if you keep doing a lot of Plan A Ben will end up in the hospital. And we won't get any sense about whether the Lexapro is getting the job done. If you can get back to doing mostly Plan C for 2 weeks, we'll get some sense about whether Ben is able to participate in Plan B once he's less irritable. I really think that's where things are at.

FATHER: Fine, fine . . . I'm back to Plan C.

MOTHER: I'll believe it when I see it.

THERAPIST: Mr. R, should we talk a little about what you can do during the next 2 weeks if your Plan A instincts are starting to kick in?

TAKING CONTROL OF THE CASE

As you now know, in the first few meetings with a child and his adult caretakers, the therapist is aggressively pursuing an understanding of the child's pathways, informally collecting information about caretakers' pathways and stressors, identifying triggers, and describing the plans framework. But the therapist is also assessing the level of hostility between the child and his adult caretakers to determine whether they are yet able to participate in Plan B discussions together. In some circumstances (e.g., when it is clear that the child and the adult are not yet able to exchange ideas without a dramatic rise in hostilities), an important role for the therapist is that of mediator or conduit between the warring parties, at least until the factions are better able to tolerate direct interactions. In such cases, the therapist explores possible solutions to conflicts between the two parties without the parties interacting directly with each other. Although this circumstance does not provide child and adult with any practice at directly talking things through, it does set the stage for some early successes with Plan B. Even when direct discussions are possible, the therapist is keeping a watchful eye on each family member's capacity for remaining engaged without becoming emotionally overloaded and remaining sensitive to moments when one family member or another may need a break from the conversation ("I think that this conversation is getting a little too hot . . . I'm thinking that we need to take a step back for a few minutes").

The therapist is also actively calculating the pace of therapy (some children and adults have very unrealistic notions about how long it can take to help people learn how to talk to each other and solve problems collaboratively), playing an active role in determining which problems should be discussed ("I'm not sure you guys are ready to deal with that problem just yet . . . I think we should pick a different one to talk about today"), and deciding which family members ought to be involved in a given discussion at any given moment ("I'd like to get everyone's ideas on this problem, but I'm starting to think that it might not be a good idea for us to do that with everyone in the room together"). On those topics where there is the potential for all hell to break loose in the therapist's office, the therapist is taking decisive action to prevent discussions from deteriorating past the point of no return, sometimes by interrupting, sometimes by asking someone to leave the office temporarily. There is nothing to be gained by watching a family discussion degenerate to the point that family members are at their worst. The therapist can gather relevant information about the factors setting the stage for deterioration well before the family hits the proverbial "brick wall."

In addition, in many cases families are involved with multiple treaters and may be receiving contradictory advice from different clinicians who have disparate notions regarding the child's difficulties. The CPS clinician must be aware of the other treatments being delivered—including pharmacotherapy—and must point out the difficulties that can occur as a by-product of receiving conflicting guidance.

PARENT: Doug's guidance counselor thinks we should be giving Doug time-outs if he blows up at home.

CLINICIAN: That's interesting advice. Does he know Doug well?

PARENT: Not really. He's been the guidance counselor at the middle school for a long time. He knows our other kids. We told him we weren't sure you would agree with his advice.

CLINICIAN: Well, he's entitled to his opinion. But why does he think a time-out would be a good idea?

PARENT: He thinks we're coddling Doug.

CLINICIAN: Does he know about the approach we've been using?

PARENT: We tried to explain it to him. He thinks it's coddling.

CLINICIAN: I'm trying to decide how important it is that we help the guidance counselor have a more accurate perception of what we're doing. Doug's not blowing up at school, right?

PARENT: Right. But the homework they're assigning is causing blowups at home.

CLINICIAN: Sounds like it might be time for us to have a school meeting so we can get everybody on the same page, especially if they're thinking that time-outs at home are a viable solution to the difficulties Doug is having doing the homework that they're assigning.

PARENT: We were hoping you'd say that.

STAYING ON TRACK

Children and their adult caretakers often have difficulty focusing on one problem at a time, or may attempt to mix many concerns into the same Plan B discussion. Under both circumstances, the discussion may collapse under the weight of manifold concerns. It is the therapist's role to make sure the discussion stays on track and focused on one concern at a time:

MOTHER: Last night was tough.

THERAPIST: What happened?

MOTHER: Toby decided at 9 pm that he needed a new video game. That we handled with Plan C . . . his father needed something at the store anyway. Plus, Toby was spending his own money.

FATHER: But that wasn't the problem. The problem came in when we got home and the video game didn't work.

THERAPIST: Uh-oh.

FATHER: Well, even that wasn't a huge deal. Except that the video game was non-refundable and I had told him at the store that I was certain the video game would work in our computer.

THERAPIST: What plan did you use then?

MOTHER: Well, my husband was ready to give Toby the money for the video game . . . you know, more Plan C. But I sort of jumped right in with Plan A at that point.

THERAPIST: OK. How come Plan A?

MOTHER: Because I wanted to make Toby explode and ruin my evening! Just kidding. We should've done Plan B. But I did end up ruining my evening.

THERAPIST: And what was the concern that led you to Plan A?

MOTHER: First, I didn't think Toby should be going to the store at 9 P.M., whether his father was going or not. I think we need to teach Toby that he can't always get what he wants the minute an idea pops into his head.

THERAPIST: I understand. I should point out that those are two separate concerns . . . and the going to the store issue was handled with Plan C, even though it's becoming clear that you guys didn't necessarily agree on handling it that way. But I'm trying to figure out your *other* concern.

MOTHER: Well, I think he has no appreciation for the value of money and I don't think we should have to pay for a video game that doesn't work.

THERAPIST: *(turning to father)* What was your position on the issue?

FATHER: Well, I thought Toby had a point . . . I mean, I did tell him I was sure it would work . . . on the other hand, I'm wasn't sure I should be covering the total expense of the video game.

THERAPIST: Sounds like you could have potentially handled the issue with Plan B . . .

MOTHER: . . . If I'd given them the chance. I know. But also, by the time we figured out that the video game didn't work, it was 10:30 at night, Toby's past his bedtime, I'm exhausted, and I'm sick of Toby not getting to bed when he's supposed to.

THERAPIST: Wow, that's a lot of problems to solve. There's three that I can count: making sure Toby knows that he can't have what he wants the minute he wants it, who should pay for the video game that didn't work, and Toby sticking to his bedtime. Even if you had attempted Plan B last night, you wouldn't have been able to solve all those problems in the same discussion. We're going to have to take them one at a time. Which of those do you guys want to tackle first?

MOTHER: Take your pick.

THERAPIST: Well, I'd suggest that we start with the Plan B discussion that came closest to taking place last night . . . the money issue . . . and then see if we have time for the others. But we probably also need to talk about what to do if one of you is ready to do Plan B and the other is bound and determined to do Plan A.

In an earlier section, we briefly discussed the therapist's role in maintaining realistic expectations regarding the pace at which family interactions can be expected to change. Along these lines, it's also the therapist's role to ensure that participants maintain perspective on the changes that have already occurred. In other words, some participants may need the therapist's assistance in reflecting on progress that's been made since treatment was initiated or need a clear definition of the concept of "progress."

MOTHER: You know, I'm starting to wonder whether all this work we're putting in is getting us anywhere. I don't even know how much progress to expect . . . I mean, we've been at this for two months now.

THERAPIST: Let's think about it a little. I can tell you what I tend to look for in terms of progress early on and we can think about how much headway we've made. I'm mindful, of course, that Matt is at the more severe end of the explosiveness spectrum.

MOTHER: Yes. And things *are* better. His explosions are shorter than they were two months ago . . .

FATHER: . . . And he's definitely blowing up less often.

THERAPIST: Well, frequency and duration of explosions are two of the things we look at in gauging progress. And it sounds like you guys feel there's been some improvement in those areas. Would you say he's not blowing up these days over some things that would have caused explosions two months ago?

FATHER: Oh, yes. We had a problem with breakfast this morning that would have been ugly two months ago . . . and we breezed right through it.

THERAPIST: That's a good sign. I also look for whether parents seem to have a good grasp of the lagging thinking skills that are contributing to their child's explosions . . . and I think you guys are pretty solid on that count. And I look for whether the parents are using Plan B—and not Plan A— whenever possible.

MOTHER: I think we're better but we still have a ways to go there.

THERAPIST: I agree. And I look for whether a child is participating in Plan B when the opportunity presents . . . I do have the sense that Matt, despite his language issues and very short fuse, is starting to see that Plan B is a way for you guys to solve some very tough problems together.

FATHER: (*looking at mother*) I would agree with that assessment as well. Although he says he hates Plan B.

THERAPIST: It's still very hard for him. I think that's all the more reason for us to be focusing our efforts on Proactive B rather than Emergency B. We encourage Proactive B for all families, but I think Plan B will be easier for all of you—not easy, easier—if you're solving predictable problems in advance.

MOTHER: We need to do better there, too.

THERAPIST: I agree. But I'd also say you have a fair amount to show for your efforts over the past two months.

MOTHER: It's helpful to think about it this way . . . but this is so hard.

THERAPIST: No question. Hard is in the cards for a while yet.

MOTHER: You'd tell us if you thought we weren't progressing as rapidly as you thought we could or if there was something else we should be doing, yes?

THERAPIST: I would.

PATHWAYS EXTENDED

As you've no doubt noticed already, Plan B incorporates many tenets of family therapy: an appreciation of the necessity of understanding maladaptive behavior within the contexts in which it occurs, an emphasis on the transactional underpinnings of maladaptive behavior, and a reluctance to designate an "identified patient." The last tenet may be a bit puzzling to some readers, as we've been quite straightforward in asserting that explosive episodes are the by-product of lacking cognitive skills. However, thus far at least—both in this book and in the early stages of therapy with a given family—we've been a little less forthcoming about the range of individuals who might be lacking those cognitive skills! Quite frankly, our tendency to focus early in treatment on the *child's* lacking cognitive skills is largely strategic. First, focusing on the child is congruent with many parents' initial expectations about what will take place in therapy. Some parents will abandon the therapeutic ship if the prevailing winds shift too rapidly from "our child is the identified patient" to "we may have some things to work on ourselves." Second, we find that focusing initially on the *child's* pathways helps us to rapidly achieve the crucial early therapeutic goal of altering adults' perceptions of a child's outbursts (once again, from goal-oriented/intentional to learning disability). Salvador Minuchin (1974) wrote of the need for a therapist to be a good salesperson for the purpose of moving a family from their original definition of the referral problem to perceiving the problem differently and more productively. Of course, every good salesperson knows that many customers cannot be rushed. Different families not only have different *needs* but also different *speeds*. But, at some point in treatment, we are clearly addressing *adult* skill deficits (when present) just as much as *child* skill deficits, and this dual focus becomes more explicit as the family becomes more comfortable with the process of therapy.

Strategy aside, Plan B requires that children and adults *listen to each other, treat each other with mutual respect, and permit and participate in the free flow of ideas*. There are a variety of factors that may interfere with these requirements. Note that while the following discussion of these factors is oriented toward family systems, as described in Chapters 7 and 8, we have applied the same concepts to other systems as well (schools, inpatient units, and residential and juvenile corrections facilities).

It is the therapist's role to point out that the parents or siblings may be struggling with some of the pathways themselves. In other words, there are some adults who have executive deficits and therefore may have difficulty anticipating problems before they occur; defining the problem; generating alternative solutions; approaching problems in an organized, systematic fashion; and so forth. Others may have language-processing issues and, as such, may have difficulty engaging in verbal give-and-take. Still others may have difficulties corresponding with the emotion regulation pathway (chronic irritability, anxiety, obsessiveness, etc.). Yet others may be very concrete, black-and-white, literal thinkers who are unable to revise their original vision of how a problem is to be solved. Those whose difficulties emanate from the social pathway may, for example, have trouble picking up on subtle or nuanced ways in which their child communicates. All of these lagging skills have the potential to make it difficult for the interaction partners to listen to each other, treat family members with mutual respect, and permit and participate in the free flow of ideas. All are grist for the therapeutic mill.

THERAPIST: Mrs. Andrews, let me know if I'm wrong about this, but I've noticed that when you and Marvin are trying to do Plan B in my office, you seem to be at a loss for words.

MRS. ANDREWS: You noticed!

THERAPIST: I did. What do you think is going on?

Mrs. Andrews: I'm always at a loss for words.

Therapist: What do you make of that?

Mrs. Andrews: Well, you know my history.

Therapist: What part of your history are you referring to?

Mrs. Andrews: The way I was treated as a child.

Therapist: Yes, I do know that part of your history. How do you think that's coming into play?

Mrs. Andrews: I'm not very confident about my own ideas.

Therapist: So this is not just a matter of your needing more practice at knowing *what to say* when you want to empathize, or define the problem, or invite David to solve the problem with you?

Mrs. Andrews: Well . . . I don't think I'm especially quick with words . . . but mostly it's that when people around me start to get heated up, I start to shut down.

Therapist: Now, you've talked about your abuse history with other therapists, yes?

Mrs. Andrews: Oh, God, yes! Too much!

Therapist: Are you thinking that it might be useful to talk with someone about it some more?

Mrs. Andrews: Absolutely not! What I need is for you to help me not shut down when people in my family get heated up. How are we going to do that?

Therapist: That's a good question. First off, I think that you have excellent instincts about how to handle David.

Mrs. Andrews: You do? Really? Thank you.

Therapist: So I think I'll keep reminding you of that. Your instincts are good. The rest, I think we'll assume, will come with time.

Mrs. Andrews: You sure?

Therapist: No, I'm not sure. But we'll operate on that assumption for the time being and then see if there's anything else we might need to work on. But I'm thinking that you're going to get a lot of practice doing Plan B in my office . . . and I think I can keep things contained enough so that you don't shut down completely. I think the more you use Plan B, the more automatic it will be and the calmer things will be over time.

Notice that, in considering and discussing adult pathways, the rules are the same. So long as we are defining the mother's difficulties as "she has an abuse history," we won't have any skills to train. If we instead identify that the mother has difficulty not shutting down, then we have skills to train.

THERAPIST: Mr. Martinez, you've been working on your anger management difficulties with a therapist for a long time, yes?

MR. MARTINEZ: Yes.

THERAPIST: And I understand that you feel it's been very helpful?

MR. MARTINEZ: Very helpful.

THERAPIST: And yet you still have a great deal of difficulty controlling your anger with Orlando, and that often prevents you from doing Plan B.

MR. MARTINEZ: He sets me off on purpose . . . he taunts me.

THERAPIST: As we've discussed, Orlando feels he's only treating you the way you've treated him for a long time. Now, that doesn't make it OK for him to treat you that way. In fact, as you know, we were able to get Orlando to stop treating you that way, even though he was skeptical that you would ever change. The problem is, every time you scream at him or criticize him, he quickly reverts back to form.

MR. MARTINEZ: Yes, that's true.

THERAPIST: I'm wondering if maybe it's time to consider whether you might benefit from other forms of treatment.

MR. MARTINEZ: Like what?

THERAPIST: Medicine.

MR. MARTINEZ: (*with a raised voice*) I'm not taking medicine just because my son treats me with disrespect!

MRS. MARTINEZ: Your son is not the only person you have trouble controlling your anger with.

MR. MARTINEZ: (*voice still raised*) My son is not the only one who treats me with disrespect!

THERAPIST: Mr. Martinez, you and I know each other pretty well at this point. We've been working on doing Plan B for a while now. It is very hard for many people to stay calm while they're doing Plan B. But Plan B—once people get the hang of it—actually helps keep people calm because they now have a road map for solving the problems that were getting them angry in the first place. But some folks—and I think this may be true of you—can't even get to Plan B because their emotions get to the problem first. I think we've seen that many times as we've tried to practice Plan B in here, yes?

MR. MARTINEZ: Yes. But only crazy people take medicine.

MRS. MARTINEZ: Your son takes medicine.

MR. MARTINEZ: He's crazy!

THERAPIST: Medicine is not just for crazy people. I'm thinking medicine could help you in two ways. First, I think it could help enhance your mood a bit. As we've discussed, you spend a lot of your time in a very irritable, agitated mood. Medicine could help with that. Second, I'm thinking medicine could help give you a longer fuse. I don't think you're crazy. I do think you could be a lot less agitated and have a longer fuse so your emotions don't beat Plan B to the problems you're trying to solve with Orlando.

MR. MARTINEZ: Look, you know I'd do just about anything to make things better with Orlando. I just don't like the idea of being on medicine. You seem to be saying that this is *my* problem.

THERAPIST: This is a *family* problem. One very irritable member of the family is already taking medicine. Another very irritable member of the family is having trouble doing Plan B and discussing things calmly. Perhaps we could help that member of the family with medicine as well. There aren't all that many things that medicine does well, but irritability is one of them. I hate to see you be so agitated and have such a short fuse when there's something that could actually be very helpful.

MR. MARTINEZ: What are the side effects?

THERAPIST: Here's what I'm thinking. Let's have you sit down with someone who prescribes medicine for adults. Now, just because you sit down with him doesn't mean you've agreed to take medicine, it just means you're getting educated about the possibilities. That's the best person to help you understand what your options are and what the side effects might be. Sound like a plan?

MR. MARTINEZ: Yes.

Sometimes an adult caretaker has already become aware of the fact that his or her own pathways may be contributing to explosive episodes. Commonly, this is revealed with a sheepish admission.

PARENT: You know, Doc, I think I may have some of these problems myself.

THERAPIST: Really . . . how so?

PARENT: I'm starting to notice that I don't have a very long fuse either.

THERAPIST: Well, that's good to know. We know that Wendy's difficulties with frustration tolerance and flexibility center on her irritability and language-processing issues. Any ideas about what might be contributing to your difficulties?

PARENT: I think I may have the irritability thing, too.

THERAPIST: Well, we should probably talk about that a little, yes?

ALTERING FAMILY COMMUNICATION PATTERNS

In his definitive book *Principles of Psychotherapy*, Dr. Irving Weiner (1975) differentiated between "process" and "content" in discussions between therapist and patients. This distinction is useful for our purposes as well. In the CPS model, *content* refers to the specifics of a given problem, or what we have previously referred to as *triggers* or *problems that have yet to be solved* (again, the list is endless, but can include homework completion, nutrition, tardiness, bedtime, curfew, and whether the content of a television show is appropriate). As we have discussed, content provides important information about events that precipitate explosive episodes and can also provide clues about the lacking cognitive skills (pathways) that may be contributing to such episodes.

At a very basic level, *process* refers to how interaction partners handled a problem or unmet expectation; as related to the CPS model, this means *whether the issue was approached with Plan A, Plan B, or Plan C*. Many families require only this very basic level of analysis of process. In such cases the therapist's role is to identify triggers and pathways, describe the plans framework, provide guidance on successful implementation of Plan B, encourage the use of Plan B instead of Plan A, and provide guidance on the various pitfalls described in Chapter 4. When this basic level of analysis fails to achieve a satisfactory outcome, therapy often moves to a more sophisticated level of process, with a stronger emphasis on general communication patterns.

In many instances, the focus is less on the pathways of the adults and more on examining communication patterns that may be making it difficult for family members to listen to each other, treat each other with mutual respect, and permit and participate in the free flow of ideas. There is no need to "reinvent the wheel" along these lines, for the rich family therapy literature is quite explicit about this type of work.

For example, in some families there may be one member who dominates conversations, preventing others from talking, minimizing others' input, shooting down ideas, talking loudly, interrupting, perhaps expressing skepticism about the value of therapy. Such a communication style not only predisposes this individual toward a Plan A approach to problems and disagreements, but is also likely to preempt the efforts of other family members to use Plan B. It's not that this person is necessarily incapable of doing Plan B at a technical level, but rather that his or her communication style and role in the system deters its use.

In some families there may be an individual who is very submissive, deferential, apparently lacking in confidence, expressing ideas (if at all) in a highly tentative fashion. The likelihood is that he or she leans heavily toward a Plan C approach to problems and disagreements. It's not that the person is incapable of doing Plan B at a technical level, but rather that his or her communication style and role in the system inhibits its use.

In many (two-adult) families, there is a natural tendency for one adult to counterbalance the behavior and style of the other, setting the stage for the classic A–C parenting combination where one adult has a strong tendency toward imposition of adult will, thereby precipitating numerous explosive episodes, and the other a strong tendency toward reducing or eliminating expectations, thereby reducing the likelihood of explosive episodes. Such an arrangement is extremely confusing to children; worse, as you already know, Plan B is not the average of Plans A and C!

Occasionally, by the way, these presentations are misleading; it is sometimes the case that an apparently domineering family member actually has very little input into actual decision making and that an apparently submissive family member is truly the eye of the hurricane. We learn about these disparities by observing (and asking questions about) who is actually participating in Plan B discussions with the child, how the solution was arrived upon, and how family members are feeling about what's transpiring in sessions.

In the following dialogue, the therapist is trying to sort through these issues. This dialogue occurred in a session that took place early in the treatment of the family of a 6-year-old boy with significant language delays. The day prior to the session, the family had endured a major explosive episode. The therapist begins the session by exploring, with the boy's parents, what transpired:

THERAPIST: Sounds like yesterday morning was tough.

FATHER: You could say it was hell.

THERAPIST: Are you guys are still suffering the after effects, or have they passed?

FATHER: They've passed but you still feel the effects.

THERAPIST: One thing is for certain, we want as little of what happened yesterday morning as possible. On that we have consensus, yes?

MOTHER: Um-hmm.

FATHER: Yeah.

THERAPIST: Do we?

FATHER: Well I don't know what story you heard, so I . . .

THERAPIST: Tell me.

FATHER: My wife told Ricky to take a shower. She said it 10, 15 times. "Take a shower." This is why I say that she gives in. He just says no and sits on the couch. So finally I said, "Ricky you are taking a shower." And I brought him upstairs, almost dragging him up, and I said, "You're taking a shower." And he wouldn't get into the shower—he's in the bathroom but he would not get in. So I wasn't gonna give in, so we started having a shouting match and my wife comes upstairs yelling, "Stop it, stop it." It's like she's worried about the neighbors. I'm like, "No, I'm not gonna give in to him." So I made him take a shower. I don't know, maybe it got out of control and maybe it didn't, but he gets his way whenever he feels like it.

THERAPIST: Would yesterday morning have been more pleasant all the way around if he had taken a shower without all the other stuff that went along with it?

FATHER: That would be ideal.

THERAPIST: Here's what I know. Giving in hasn't served you well. But screaming hasn't served you well either. There's got to be another way. There's got to be a way to see if we can actually make something happen without all the screaming. If screaming at Ricky was going to work, it would have worked a long time ago. A *very* long time ago. (*looking at father*) Let me ask you an important question. Your wife is the one who told Ricky to take a shower. But how important was it to *you* that he take a shower?

FATHER: When he pees in his bed in the middle of the night, he just stinks, so he had to take a shower.

THERAPIST: Right. But on a scale of 1 to 10, with 10 being "This is absolutely critical" and 1 being . . .

FATHER: I see what you're getting at. I wouldn't have made him take a shower.

THERAPIST: You wouldn't have made him take a shower?

MOTHER: I was just gonna say that. There was no way that he would have had him take a shower. It was me. He was doing it for me.

THERAPIST: (*to father*) Well . . . you inherited her Plan A, didn't you?

FATHER: It's been a long-standing problem. She tells him to do something and she doesn't enforce it. If I'm with him and I tell him to do something, sometimes I have to use some yelling or take things away, but he usually does it. But when she tells him to do something she doesn't stand behind it.

THERAPIST: (*to mother*) So you start out using Plan A and tell Ricky to do something and he balks and you tell him again and he balks again and 15 times later you're still telling him to do the same thing.

MOTHER: Right.

THERAPIST: (*to father*) Eventually, your fuse is lit. You're sitting there listening to this and you're thinking, my God, it's 15 times now. You're thinking, *she* can't get him to do it . . . *I'll* get him to do it.

FATHER: Right, exactly.

THERAPIST: (*to father*) At that moment you have inherited your wife's Plan A on an issue that you didn't care much about in the first place. But then it starts getting messier with you and Ricky. (*to mother*) And then you revert from Plan A to Plan C and you're saying, "You know what, it just isn't worth it. Just leave it alone."

MOTHER: Right.

THERAPIST: So there's two points at which you guys disagree with each other. First you disagree over how to handle a problem with Ricky. That's on the front end. Then you disagree once it gets messy, but in the exact opposite way: Mrs. S, that's when you're ready to use Plan C, and Mr. S, that's when you refuse to quit and pick up with Plan A where your wife left off. Problem is, you guys are acting like there's only two options: you can either have a war or you can give in. But those two options have only gotten you a lot of therapy, a lot of medicine, and not a lot of progress with Ricky.

MOTHER: That's true.

THERAPIST: There's a good reason that those two options haven't gotten you very far. Neither fixes the problem. Clearly everybody felt bad about what happened yesterday. (*to father*) In your mind, what's the worst thing that happened in the whole episode?

FATHER: Disagreeing with my wife. I was kinda hoping that someday maybe we'd be on the same page. She started the shower thing and she wouldn't stick to her guns. As soon as Ricky clearly wouldn't do it, she just gave in.

MOTHER: I do a lot of Plan C.

THERAPIST: You do a lot of Plan C, but you do a lot of Plan C after you've done Plan A and that's what drives your husband crazy because that's capitulating. See, when you start out with A and end up doing C, that's giving in. But when you *start out* doing C you're saying, "I know my kid. I know what he can and can't do. I know what we're working on right now. I know what we're not working on right now. We're not working on this right now. That's Plan C. I'm not saying a word."

MOTHER: That's where my husband was on the shower.

THERAPIST: Right. By the way, especially early on, you'll get no fight from me if you're using Plan C on something. If you guys come in next week and say, "We just decided that brushing your teeth is being handled with Plan C," I'll say, "Congratulations, fantastic, great idea—don't even bring it up, at least not yet." If you come in and say that brushing your teeth is being handled with Plan A and we fought with him all week and we hate each other now and our daughter's upset and Ricky's been hit with a belt because we used Plan A, then I'll say you shouldn't have used Plan A.

MOTHER: So just don't even mention it?

THERAPIST: If you're doing Plan C. I'm actually thinking there are many things you might normally want him to do that we aren't going to ask him to do for a while in the service of fewer explosions. You've seen the damage Plan A does to this family. Reducing explosions has to be our top priority for a while. So we need to stay away from Plan A. But we mostly need to get you guys good at Plan B. That's where you guys come together.

FATHER: We're not good at that yet.

THERAPIST: Nobody gets good at Plan B instantaneously. It's hard. Let's think about what the shower episode would have looked like if you were doing Plan B, shall we?

FATHER: Sure.

THERAPIST: Plan B starts with empathy. What would you guys have said to empathize?

MOTHER: "You don't want to take a shower?"

THERAPIST: Sounds good to me. Then what?

MOTHER: "But I want you to take a shower."

THERAPIST: Not so fast. Do we know why he doesn't want to take a shower? What his concern is?

MOTHER: (*looking at husband*) Do you?

FATHER: He doesn't like the way it feels.

THERAPIST: For real? He doesn't like the way it feels?

FATHER: Yeah. He's told me that before.

THERAPIST: OK, so how would we get that concern on the table?

FATHER: I'd just say, "You don't like the way the shower feels."

THERAPIST: Good. Then what?

MOTHER: So then we'd say, "But we want you to take a shower"?

THERAPIST: Well, I'd say that's not a very specific concern, either. Why do you want him to take a shower?

FATHER: Because he stinks from peeing in his bed.

THERAPIST: Let's get that concern on the table. What would you say?

FATHER: I'd say, "But we'd like to clean you up because you smell like pee."

THERAPIST: OK. Last step?

MOTHER: The invitation!

THERAPIST: Good. How would you invite him to solve the problem with you?

MOTHER: I'd say, "How can we work that out?"

THERAPIST: Great. Would Ricky have any ideas?

MOTHER: (*looking at husband*) I don't know.

THERAPIST: Do you guys have any ideas?

FATHER: He could take a bath.

THERAPIST: Does he mind taking baths?

FATHER: No, he likes baths.

THERAPIST: He likes baths? I'm confused. If he likes baths, why are we telling him to take a shower?

MOTHER: (*looking at husband*) I don't think we've ever thought about it.

THERAPIST: So if you say, "It's time for a bath," he doesn't balk?

MOTHER: Well, maybe he balks a little because he's in the middle of something, but he goes.

THERAPIST: Wow. Well, one of the things we need to spend some time on is the specific triggers that cause a lot of blowups. But we also need to start having these conversations ahead of time—you know, proactively—so we're not stuck trying to solve a problem in the heat of the moment.

We're going to start knocking off one problem at a time. But here's the pep talk: give yourselves a month or two to get good at it. Give him a month or two to get good at it. Don't expect Plan B to change your life overnight because he's a complicated kid, and this is a family that's in pretty desperate straits, and you don't fix that in a day. You fix it slowly but surely. Having said that, it may fix a whole lot faster than you think.

MOTHER: Thank you. That's what we needed, someone to even just say this.

THERAPIST: Good. He's a great kid.

MOTHER: Oh, we know that.

THERAPIST: When the stage is set for him to be a great kid, he is a great kid. When the stage is not set for him to be a great kid, you see him at his worst. Plan B sets the stage for him to be at his best and has you guys on the same page.

When a family member is dominating conversations, it is the therapist's role to set the stage for others to speak, sometimes by interrupting or asking that the family member withhold his or her comments for a while so that others may speak ("Mr. Sanchez, I think you've done a very nice job of letting us know where you stand on this issue. . . . Now I think it would be good to hear from others about where they stand"). When a family member blames another for problems that are really more reflective of relationship issues, it is the therapist's role to provide direct feedback along these lines: "Mr. Taylor, so long as you think that your difficulties with your son are his fault, I don't think we're going to get very far." When a family member seems reluctant to speak, the therapist's role is to gently encourage that person to express him- or herself, while remaining sensitive to any factors or pathways that may be inhibiting such expression ("Maribel, I'm getting the sense that you have some ideas of your own on this topic . . . I think it would be very good for us to hear what you're thinking"). If the therapist has effectively established rapport with each family member, it should be possible to deliver this feedback and steer the ship in a different direction without a member of the crew jumping overboard.

When a family member is minimizing the ideas of another, it's the therapist's role to provide a counterbalance.

ADOLESCENT: If you guys [the parents] think I spend too much money, then why don't I get a job so I can stop asking you for money!

PARENT: That is the most ridiculous idea I've ever heard.

THERAPIST: Actually, I think it might be good to keep all our options open . . . Maribel getting a job might be an idea worth thinking about.

In some families, the affect of one or more members is so intense, and emotions on such a hair trigger, that the instant a difficult topic is broached, listening, mutual respect, and a free flow of ideas becomes impossible. The therapist, of course, must decide whether the topic is yet in the "discussable" range. But often, when family members are unable to speak directly to each other, the therapist can do the talking for one of the members so as to "take the affective head off the beer."

FATHER: I'd like to spend today talking about why Marvin is doing no homework.

MARVIN: (*instantaneously agitated*) Who said I'm doing no homework?

FATHER: Well, I don't see you doing it at home, so I'm assuming you're not doing your homework. All I'm seeing is you getting completely stressed out every Sunday night because you don't have your homework done.

MARVIN: (*still screaming*) I do it at school, you f——ing moron!

FATHER: Well, you must not be doing it all at school because you're still getting stressed out every Sunday night and I don't feel like living that way.

MARVIN: (looking at therapist) I can't talk to this f——ing idiot! (*through gritted teeth*) He makes me so f——ing mad!

THERAPIST: Well, I actually don't know if you all are ready to talk about this right now, but I think your father is just saying he'd like to see if there's a way to help you be less stressed out about homework.

MARVIN: They can send me to a different school.

FATHER: We're not sending you to a different school.

MARVIN: (*agitated again*) Why not, you fat jerk?

THERAPIST: Marvin, what kind of a different school are you talking about?

MARVIN: A lot of my friends go to a private school, and . . .

FATHER: There is no way he's going to a private school. What school he goes to has nothing to do with . . .

MARVIN: (*screaming*) If he won't let me talk I won't stay in here!

THERAPIST: (*to father*) I think that you're often saying that you wish Marvin would tell you what's going on in his head, and I think that he was about to tell you, so I think we should listen.

FATHER: Fine. I'm listening.

THERAPIST: Marvin, what were you going to say?

MARVIN: He won't interrupt?

THERAPIST: (*looking at father*) He won't interrupt you.

MARVIN: I can't stand the kids at my school. I hate them. They're all punks or into drugs, they make it hard to learn, and I'm stressed out all day at school being with them. I want to go to a different school.

THERAPIST: And you have a certain different school in mind?

MARVIN: Yes, it's a private school, a lot of my friends go there, and . . .

FATHER: And it costs $7,000 a year!

MARVIN: God-dammit, *I'm* talking!

THERAPIST: Mr. L, I promise you'll get your concerns on the table. Right now, we're trying to get Marvin's concerns on the table.

FATHER: I thought it was a relevant fact.

THERAPIST: It may well be, but not yet. Marvin, keep going.

MARVIN: That's it. I want to go to a different school, and these morons won't let me.

THERAPIST: So let me make sure I've got it right. You hate the kids at your school, you feel like they make it difficult for you to learn, you want to go somewhere else. Yes?

MARVIN: Yes.

THERAPIST: (*turning to parents*) And you guys have some concerns about Marvin going to this private school, yes?

FATHER: Yes. It costs $7,000 a year and we're not sure that the school can meet all of Marvin's needs.

MARVIN: You drive a $30,000 car! And you can't afford to spend $7,000 on me?

FATHER: The car is paid for. Private school is not paid for. And I have a philosophical objection to paying tax money in my town for him to go to public school and spending another $7,000 for him to go to some private school! That's not the way the world works, and it's time for Marvin to start living in the . . .

THERAPIST: I think that your concern about what the private school costs is already on the table.

FATHER: (*turning to mother*) I can't do this! This is bullsh——t! Plan B is bullsh——t.

MOTHER: (*to father*) I know this is hard for you.

FATHER: (*pointing at Marvin*) And he's not even talking! We still don't know why he won't do his homework!

THERAPIST: I think he told us why he has trouble doing his homework.

FATHER: Why, what did he say?

THERAPIST: He said the kids at school are making it hard for him to learn.

FATHER: How is that affecting his homework? It has nothing to do with his homework!

MARVIN: (*jumping out of his seat*) I cannot stay in the room with this a—— hole!

THERAPIST: (*to Marvin*) Marvin, you're doing a very good job of expressing yourself today, but I'd like to try something. I'm going to do the talking for you for a while. You don't have to talk. If I get something wrong, you correct me. If your father says something you object to, let's see if I can help him understand where you're coming from. That OK?

MARVIN: (*sitting down*) Fine.

THERAPIST: It makes some sense to me that if Marvin is extremely unhappy with his circumstances at school that might make it hard for him to do his homework. I think that's what he's saying.

FATHER: Why didn't he say that? Why does he need you to do his talking for him?

THERAPIST: Well, I think he did say that. I think that the way in which you're responding makes it hard for him to talk directly to you. So I'll talk for him. You don't upset me as much as you upset him.

FATHER: So now I'm the problem!

THERAPIST: No, the way your family communicates is the problem. As a member of the family, you are part of the problem. You see, it doesn't really matter what we talk about . . . the problems you guys have in talking to each other come up regardless of the topic.

FATHER: He's not doing his homework and now I'm the problem! (*turning to wife*) This is why we're coming here? This is what I'm paying for?

THERAPIST: You're coming here so you guys can learn how to talk to each other. I wonder if we could get back to the homework issue.

FATHER: Fine by me.

THERAPIST: Mrs. L, I wonder if you'd like to say anything?

MOTHER: Well, I know this is very hard for Marvin and my husband. But I do think Marvin is trying very hard to talk.

FATHER: (*to therapist*) Great! Now you've got her taking his side, too!

THERAPIST: This isn't about sides. I'm trying to help you guys talk to each other. You both have valid concerns about the homework issue. Marvin hates the kids at his school and thinks that's why he's so stressed out and having trouble getting his work done. You don't have $7,000 for him to go to a different school and are concerned that the different school might not be able to meet his needs. I think you guys can talk about that. But I want to make the point that the problem won't get solved unless *both* sets of concerns are on the table . . . Marvin's *and* yours.

FATHER: But why does he need you to talk for him?

THERAPIST: Because when he talks, you tell him he's not talking. And because, I must say, it's not clear that you're hearing what he's saying. That makes it extremely difficult for him to keep talking.

Q & A

What are the most common difficulties you see families encountering in implementing this model?

Many adults aren't aware that they have other options besides Plan A. It's the therapist's role to help them become aware of their other options. Once aware of these options, many adults still have difficulty recognizing when they are using Plan A. It's the therapist's role to help them become aware of their Plan A tendencies and begin using other options (Plan B) when they wish to pursue their expectations. Many adults believe that CPS is a very permissive approach to discipline and that Plan B means letting the child get his way. It's up to the therapist to help adults understand that there is nothing permissive about the CPS model (remember, adults are pursuing their expectations and setting limits whether they're using Plan A or Plan B), and that the problem isn't solved until the adult's (and child's) concerns have been satisfactorily addressed. Many adults just need lots of practice at Plan B; that, of course, is one of the primary activities during therapy sessions.

I've been taught that it's important for parents to be consistent with each other in front of the child so the child can't do any "splitting." So what advice do you give parents if one is using Plan A on an issue and the other disagrees?

We think explosions are far more destructive to families than parents disagreeing in front of their children. So if two parents *share the same concern* and one is handling the concern with Plan A and about to cause an explosion, we have no qualms about telling the other parent to intervene (quickly) so as to initiate Plan B and head off an explosion. That's not "splitting" or "undermining," that's just good teamwork. Of course, in a subsequent session, we'd want to make sure that we clarified why the first adult decided that Plan A was the best approach to the problem and remind him or her that any problem that can be handled with Plan A can also be handled with Plan B.

Life is a bit more interesting if one parent is using Plan A and the other is using Plan C, for this suggests that the parents are not yet in agreement about whether they should be putting an adult concern on the table. The therapist's role here is to help the parents achieve a consensus on whether the concern is actually worth pursuing and to encourage them to have such discussions prior to handling a problem with Plan A, Plan B, or Plan C. If one parent thinks a concern is worth putting on the table and the other parent disagrees, it's fine to tell a child that the conversation may have to be delayed until the parents have had a chance to consult with one another.

In some of the preceding dialogues, the therapist was meeting only with the parents; in others, only with the child; and in others, with parents and the child together. How much does the child take part in sessions? How do you decide when to have the child participate and when not to?

Pragmatics and goals dictate who we're meeting with at any given time. If we feel that establishing a strong bond with the child is a therapeutic priority, we might meet with the child first (without the caretakers) at the beginning of early sessions. By contrast, if we feel caretakers need a great deal of support and encouragement, we might meet with the caretakers at the beginning of each session. If we want to make sure that the child and caretakers have ample opportunities to practice Plan B under the supervision of the therapist, then having child and caretakers in the office together becomes a high priority. Although CPS is a family therapy model, as we've said elsewhere we don't believe it makes sense to meet with all family members for the entirety of every session. Early on, we'd rather set the stage for successful implementation of Plan B by strategically meeting with the conflicting parties separately prior to having them attempt to talk together.

Chapter 6

Skills Trained with Plan B

As noted earlier, there are several specific cognitive skills necessary for participating in Plan B discussions, and a variety of additional skills that are central to managing frustration in general. In this chapter, we focus on the manner by which the CPS model trains these skills. While basic Plan B is effective at training many lacking cognitive skills, other skills may require slight modifications to Plan B or some augmentative forms of training. It goes without saying that, although our focus in this chapter is on skills *children* may be lacking, we often find the same skills lacking (and requiring remediation) in adult caretakers. While research has shown the CPS model to significantly reduce oppositional behavior, improve parent–child interactions, and reduce parenting stress (see Chapter 9), support for the skills-training dimension of the model is, at this writing, anecdotal.

SKILLS NEEDED FOR PLAN B

Let's begin by discussing elementary skills that are necessary for participating in Plan B discussions. At a very basic level, Plan B requires that participants have the capacity to *identify and articulate their concerns so as to identify the problem to be solved, consider possible solutions, and reflect on the feasibility and likely outcomes of solutions and the degree to which they are mutually satis-*

factory. As a child and his adult caretakers first begin attempting Plan B discussions, it's important for the clinician to assess whether the lack of these skills in either party is interfering with successful participation.

Identifying and Articulating Concerns

Many explosive children—especially (but not always) those whose difficulties stem from the language-processing pathway—have difficulty verbalizing what it is that they are frustrated about. Our situational analysis can be very useful here, for it permits us to proactively home in on situations or triggers that are routinely frustrating the child and helps us to be highly specific in training an initial pragmatic vocabulary. For example, if a child with sensory hypersensitivities was having difficulty verbalizing the fact that the tags in his clothing were bothersome, and if this trigger was accounting for a meaningful number of explosive episodes, then training a vocabulary that permits the child to articulate this problem should be worthwhile, beginning with, "The tags in my clothing are bugging me." It would make sense to have a Proactive Plan B discussion (perhaps in the therapist's office) about the need for a way to verbalize this frustration, with some resolution regarding actual wording. Here's how that might sound:

THERAPIST: (*modeling empathy*) I've heard that the labels in your clothing bug you a lot.

CHILD: Yup.

THERAPIST: (*modeling more empathy*) And I've heard that it's not so easy for you to say that the labels are bugging you.

CHILD: It's not?

PARENT: (*modeling problem definition*) Well, I told Dr. Samuels that when you're frustrated about the labels you sometimes say some words that aren't very nice.

CHILD: Oh, yeah.

THERAPIST: (*modeling invitation*) So, I think your mom and dad know how much the labels bug you . . . but we wish we could come up with a way for you to say that the labels are bugging you without you saying words that aren't very nice. Can you think of any ideas for how we could do that?

At this point, the discussion would center on agreeing upon the words the child could use to signal that a label is bothersome. Naturally, if we are secure in a "children do well if they can" mentality, then we would assume that if the child already knew more appropriate words he'd already be using them. So there's a good chance that generic assistance such as "use your words" is unlikely to help, and that instead the child will need some suggestions. Note that in merely raising the issue, a possible phrase ("The label is bugging me") has already been introduced.

Of course, one Proactive Plan B discussion is unlikely to suffice in training the articulation of concerns. It's a pretty sure bet that the child will need some "in-the-moment" reminders as a follow-up to this discussion:

CHILD: I hate this shirt! It sucks!

ADULT: Uh-oh . . . looks like the label is bugging you.

Also note that the adult isn't saying "Don't forget what we agreed on yesterday" or "You can't talk to me that way," because these aren't specific enough reminders of the new vocabulary. Also note that the adult isn't saying "Can you think of a better way to say that?" How rapidly will a child begin to reliably use his new vocabulary? That varies . . . certainly not after only one trial. But we fully expect that after sufficient reminders the child will eventually come forth with "The label is bugging me!"

We also find it useful to train a vocabulary that can be applied cross-situationally. For example, "The label in my shirt is bugging me" would really only be applicable to situations in which labels in clothing are bothersome. But phrases like "Gimme a minute," "I can't talk about that right now," "I need help," "Something is bothering me," and "I don't know what to do" can be used in a wider range of circumstances. These phrases would be trained in the same manner as the more specific vocabulary illustrated above. In other words, the role of the surrogate frontal lobe is to use Proactive Plan B to help generate a set of common expressions that can be used across situations and then to remind the child of his new vocabulary.

Now, sometimes children have difficulty articulating their concern because they *don't know* what their concern is. Since it will be impossible to proceed with Plan B until the child's concern is on the table, it's important to figure it out. Here's an example of what a Proactive Plan B discussion would sound like in the therapist's office if this were the case:

THERAPIST: (*basic empathy*) I understand you don't want to come in for our family meetings anymore.

CHILD: Right.

THERAPIST: (*reassurance, then attempting to clarify the child's concern*) We're not saying you have to keep coming. But how come you don't want to come in anymore?

CHILD: I don't know.

THERAPIST: Hmm. Should we see if your mom can help out here?

CHILD: She just tells me I have to come.

THERAPIST: Well, I was wondering if your mom had any ideas about why you don't want to keep coming. (*looking at mother*) Mom, do you have any ideas?

MOTHER: To tell you the honest truth, I'm not sure.

THERAPIST: OK. Well, I can think of a few reasons why some other kids I've worked with didn't want to keep coming. Maybe one of these reasons is true for you. Would you like to hear them?

CHILD: OK.

THERAPIST: Some of the kids I've worked with didn't like sitting in the car a long time to get here. Is that true for you?

CHILD: No. It doesn't take us very long to get here.

THERAPIST: OK. Some other kids didn't feel very comfortable talking about times when they and their parents had trouble getting along. What about that one?

CHILD: No. I don't care about that.

THERAPIST: Hmm. Well, some kids have something they'd rather do than be here. Is that it?

CHILD: Yep.

THERAPIST: (*back to empathy*) Ah, there's something else you want to be doing besides being here. What is it?

CHILD: Well, it's not that I don't like being here. It's just that I wanted to go out for the basketball team, and practices don't get over until 5:30.

THERAPIST: (*reempathizing yet again*) You want to go out for the basketball team and the time of the practices would interfere with you coming here.

CHILD: Right.

Of course, the Plan B discussion would continue with the remaining steps, now that the child's concern has been specifically defined.

In cases where the child is having difficulty communicating concerns that are routinely frustrating, we have found it helpful for the therapist, in collaboration with the child and his adult caretakers, to generate a list of these common concerns. Remember that although explosive episodes often appear to be random and unpredictable to adults, thinking in situational terms reminds us that they are highly predictable and precipitated by a few common triggers or concerns. Thus, creating a list of common concerns or triggers can usually be easily accomplished. For example, in the case of one adolescent who became extremely frustrated when he was unable to articulate the source of his frustration, a Proactive Plan B discussion was used to generate a list of common concerns, including changes in plan, thinking people were mad at him, feeling misunderstood, feeling not listened to, being told what to do, being bored, and being annoyed. Whenever the boy became agitated, his parents would remind him of his new vocabulary by retrieving the list, reciting the items, and asking if any of the items applied to his current frustration. After 2 weeks of this intervention, he began telling the parents what was frustrating him without the aid of the list (and without the explosive episodes that accompanied his frustration at being unable to identify his concerns).

Considering Possible Solutions

Generating alternative solutions is one of the key skills being facilitated by the invitation, where child and adult are brainstorming potential solutions that are intended to take both concerns into account. When children are unable to generate any solutions (sometimes this is because the child has bona fide difficulties originating solutions; in other circumstances, it's because the child has never been permitted the *opportunity* to demonstrate a capacity for originating solutions), we encourage the surrogate frontal lobe to generate solutions, but always in a suggestive rather than a definitive manner ("Well, here's a possibility . . . let me know what you think of this idea"). We find that after experiencing numerous repetitions of an adult generating alternative solutions, children's capacities for the same skill begin to develop. Of course, if the adult caretakers have poorly developed solution-generating skills, the likely mechanism for skill enhancement will be the therapist modeling generating alternative solutions.

In some cases, simply modeling the process of brainstorming solutions will not be sufficient to train the skill. In these cases, we often find it useful to provide children and adults with a simple framework for generating solutions.

It may be hard to believe, but it turns out that the vast majority of solutions to problems encountered by human beings falls into one of three general categories:

1. Ask for help.
2. Meet halfway/give a little.
3. Do it a different way.

So we often train this framework to lend structure to the solution-generating process. This framework can be very helpful to children with significant language delays, for it simplifies the language of problem solving (and can be accomplished through pictures rather than words). The framework can also be helpful to black-and-white thinkers who have difficulty envisioning solutions that differ from whatever solution they originally configured, as well as to children and adults who, perhaps due to disorganized or impulsive thinking or poor working memory, become easily overwhelmed by the mere prospect of contemplating possible solutions (and their outcomes) or by the universe of potential solutions. Here's what practicing the new framework might look like in the therapist's office:

THERAPIST: I've noticed that you guys often seem to get stuck after you've figured out what the problem is. You know what each other's concerns are, but you're not exactly sure how to go about solving the problem. That's where you get stuck.

CHILD: Yeah, that's because we both stink at it!

ADULT: Hey, I'll admit it. I get started OK but then I don't seem to have any good ideas for solutions.

THERAPIST: I think I have some ideas that might help get you guys started. There really are only three different types of solutions that people tend to use to fix problems. They either "ask for help," "meet halfway," or "do it a different way." So, for instance, if you and your sister both wanted to play Nintendo at the same time, which option makes the most sense?

CHILD: I don't know.

ADULT: Meet halfway, right? Like each use it for 10 minutes.

THERAPIST: And what if you wanted to go for ice cream after this appointment, but the place you usually go was closed?

CHILD: Go somewhere else?

THERAPIST: Sounds good. That would be "doing it a different way." And how about if you can't figure out your math homework?

CHILD: Ask for help.

THERAPIST: Excellent. If you guys are getting stuck, you might want to try using those three options as a road map: ask for help, meet halfway, do it a different way.

After this framework is trained using Proactive Plan B, it can be invoked whenever the process of considering possible solutions is initiated (whether using Proactive or Emergency Plan B). Here's how the framework would sound if an adult were practicing at home using Proactive Plan B:

ADULT: (*empathy*) I've noticed that you've been very unhappy when I pick you up at school lately. What's up?

CHILD: It's embarrassing to have you pick me up at school. No one else has to get picked up by their parents.

ADULT: (*reempathizing, then reassuring, then defining the problem, then inviting*) It's embarrassing to you for me to pick you up at school. I'm not saying I have to pick you up at school. I'm just concerned that you won't get to your violin lesson on time if I don't pick you up. Can you think of how we can solve that problem?

CHILD: No. I don't know.

ADULT: (*categorizing potential solutions*) Let's see if what Dr. Sam taught us will help. I don't know if "asking for help" will solve this problem. I can't think of how we would "meet halfway or give a little" on this one. I'm thinking this is one where we'd try to "do it a different way." What do you think?

CHILD: Yeah.

ADULT: (*now ready to brainstorm*) Can you think of a different way for us to get you to your violin lesson on time without me embarrassing you by picking you up at school?

CHILD: We could ask Mrs. Perkins to make my violin lesson later. Then I could take the bus home from school and you could take me to my lesson after I got home.

Naturally, this Plan B discussion would continue until a feasible, realistic, mutually satisfactory solution was agreed upon. Notice that the process enables the child to learn through active involvement in the generation of the solution as opposed to being the passive beneficiary of adult ingenuity.

Reflecting on the Likely Outcomes of Solutions and the Degree to Which They Are Feasible and Mutually Satisfactory

Many children have difficulty projecting solutions into the future so as to consider likely outcomes; others may also have difficulty focusing on whether potential solutions are feasible and mutually satisfactory (i.e., whether the solutions under consideration are truly realistic and address both concerns). It is sometimes necessary to augment Plan B by having the adult perform the task of anticipating and describing the likely outcomes of the solutions that have been generated ("Well, here's what I think will happen if we choose that solution . . . and here's what I think it will look like if we choose the second option . . . which of those outcomes do you think would work the best?"). After multiple repetitions, we anticipate that the child will ultimately improve at the skill of evaluating likely outcomes. No matter how many Plan B repetitions this requires, we know of no faster way to train this crucial cognitive skill.

On a related note, in many instances adults lose faith in Plan B because the child has *failed to follow through* on an agreed-upon solution. In fact, as mentioned earlier, this is usually the sign of an unrealistic solution or one that failed to adequately address the child's concern. We find that, in most instances, one of the two parties involved wasn't actually capable of delivering on what he or she had agreed to. Remember, Plan B isn't an exercise in wishful thinking . . . it's the hard work of helping child and adult achieve mutually satisfactory and doable solutions. As you'd expect, it's the therapist's role to express skepticism (when warranted) about solutions that don't seem to fall into the doable range. In doing so, the therapist is training adult and child in the crucial skill of projecting solutions into the future and reflecting upon their likely outcomes.

MOTHER: Tom won't do the solution he agreed to.

THERAPIST: Uh-oh. Tell me.

MOTHER: Well, we had a Proactive Plan B discussion with him about homework this week. We were very proud of ourselves. He agreed that he'd do his homework every day at 4 o'clock. So we have this conversation with him on Monday night. On Tuesday . . . Tuesday! . . . he didn't get to it until 7 o'clock! He didn't start his homework once at 4 o'clock the whole week! What's the point of doing Plan B if he's not going to do what he agreed to?

THERAPIST: Well, there is no point in doing Plan B if people don't do what they agree to. Tom, any thoughts about what happened?

TOM: (*hanging his head*) No. I don't know.

THERAPIST: I have some thoughts.

FATHER: We'd love to hear them.

THERAPIST: Usually when people don't follow through on an agreed-upon solution, it's because it was an unrealistic solution.

MOTHER: What does that mean?

THERAPIST: It means that, given what we know about Tom, I have some serious doubts about whether he can actually start his homework at 4 o'clock. I just can't see it happening. So if he can't do it, we're still looking for a realistic solution.

FATHER: But he agreed to it!

THERAPIST: Yes . . . he really shouldn't have. Mrs. Costello, you've always been home with Tom at homework time . . . do you really think he can start his homework at 4 o'clock?

MOTHER: Well he did agree to.

THERAPIST: Yes, I understand . . . but do you think he can do it? Reliably?

MOTHER: (*laughing nervously*) No . . . he never has. He really does seem to need more downtime than that after school.

THERAPIST: Since the solution wasn't realistic and probably didn't really address Tom's concerns, then you guys probably shouldn't have agreed to the solution either.

FATHER: So what does that mean . . . he doesn't have to do his homework?

THERAPIST: That would be Plan C. And he did do his homework. But I think we're looking for a more realistic solution than the one you all first agreed to and one that does a better job of addressing Tom's concern. I'm delighted that you handled this issue with Plan B . . . it's just that we need to make sure that Plan B isn't simply an exercise in wishful thinking.

In other instances, adults trip up on the fact that the child doesn't seem to *care* about their concern. Here's what this might sound like:

MOTHER: (*empathizing*) I've noticed that, when you have an accident in your underpants, the only person you want to have clean you is Daddy.

CHILD: Yup.

MOTHER: (*defining the problem*) The thing is, Daddy isn't always home when you have an accident, and he can't always come home from work to clean you up.

CHILD: I don't care. I'll wait until he gets home.

MOTHER: (*defining the problem further*) I know you're willing to wait until he gets home, but we don't want you sitting around in dirty underwear for hours. It must be uncomfortable, it's bad for your skin, and it's kind of stinky for us.

CHILD: I don't care. I don't mind.

It's worth pointing out that, in this brief dialogue, the child's concern has yet to be well defined. But many adults worry that the child's lack of regard for *their* concern spells doom for Plan B. Not so. The child doesn't have to "own" the adult's concern for Plan B to proceed . . . he merely needs to take the adult's concern into account so that mutually satisfactory solutions can be discussed. So now let's go back to the unsavory issue of soiled underwear to see how the child's lack of ownership of the adults' concern might be handled:

MOTHER: (*reempathizing, redefining the problem, and inviting*) I know you don't mind. But I mind. Remember, we're trying to come up with a solution that will work well for both of us. And you sitting around in dirty underwear for hours doesn't work for me. I think we can find a way to solve this problem that will work well for both of us. So can we try again?

In still other instances, the child doesn't seem to be aware (or may appear not to care) that his solution hasn't addressed both concerns. Often, the child will simply remain stuck on an initial solution that only addressed his concern. While conventional wisdom could lead us to conclude that the child is "stubborn" or "controlling," we are, of course, instead likely to view the child as challenged in the skill of perspective taking. The adult response should be fairly similar to the above dialogue: "Curt, I know that solution would make you happy, but it wouldn't make me very happy. Let's try to think of a solution that would make both of us happy."

We are often asked what we do when two parties cannot reach a mutually satisfactory solution when attempting Plan B. Often, as discussed in Chapter

4, it is because there are two *solutions* rather than two *concerns* on the table. Once again, "dueling solutions" are unlikely to set the stage for successful resolution of a problem. Sometimes—and this is quite common in the course of human affairs—the two parties have to take a break from discussions so as to lower the heat and provide an opportunity for more reflection. In fairly rare instances, a mutually satisfactory solution is unreachable because child or adult is not yet stable enough to participate in Plan B. In such instances, it may be necessary to hold off on Plan B and aggressively pursue stabilization, often through use of Plan C and/or medication.

Which brings us to an important topic that we've neglected thus far. There are some children (and adults) who simply will not be able to participate in Plan B discussions without aid of pharmacological intervention. Those who have an extraordinarily limited capacity for tolerating frustration may explode before the calming effects of Plan B can kick in. If the "short fuse" is attributable to disorganized thinking, hyperactivity, or poor impulse control, stimulant medications are often the agents of first choice. If the poor tolerance for frustration is a by-product of irritability or obsessiveness, selective serotonin reuptake inhibitor (SSRI) antidepressants are often the agents of first choice. And if true mania or severe mood instability are implicated, then mood-stabilizing agents (such as atypical antipsychotics) may be indicated. It is worth noting that medication does not train lacking thinking skills; it merely makes such training more possible. In dedicating only one paragraph in this book to medication, we do not wish to diminish its importance in the treatment of some explosive children. On the other hand, we have seen far too many children placed on large numbers and high doses of medication because of the failure to consider cognitive factors that were contributing to their difficulties and therefore the failure to consider the potential benefits of psychosocial treatment. Even when pharmacotherapy is indicated and effective, we tend to be quite concerned about a child's long-term prognosis if the pharmacotherapy is not augmented with the teaching of lacking cognitive skills.

TRAINING OTHER SKILLS CENTRAL TO MANAGING FRUSTRATION

Now that we have discussed the teaching of basic skills necessary for participating in Plan B discussions, let's turn to consideration of a variety of additional skills embedded within each of the pathways that might be needed to help children manage frustration in general. Note that basic Plan B would train many of these additional skills, whereas others require some modification to Plan B or augmentive skills training.

Executive Skills

Improving many executive skills can be facilitated through the use of basic Plan B. You may have noticed that several executive skills were, in fact, already discussed in the preceding section. For example, when adults help a child define a problem, use hindsight to reflect on past solutions and their outcomes, and use forethought to predict likely outcomes of potential solutions, they are training more organized, planful (nonimpulsive) thinking. In fact, Proactive Plan B (anticipating and solving a problem before it happens again) is by its very nature planful and nonimpulsive.

Basic Plan B is effective at improving a child's capacity for shifting cognitive set as well. As previously defined in Chapter 1, shifting cognitive set refers to the speed and efficiency with which an individual is able to shift from the rules and expectations of one situation to those of another. There are basically two ways to help a child shift set. One is to *demand* that he shift set: "Jose, just in case you didn't notice, science class began 2 minutes ago . . . get your materials out for science and get to work . . . *now.*" That would be Plan A. The other is to *help* him shift set. If demanding that he shift set is precipitating explosive episodes, and if he is routinely and predictably having difficulty shifting set, we strongly suggest the latter approach. Because most shifts in cognitive set are highly predictable (moving from class to class, waking up, turning off the TV to come to dinner), Proactive Plan B is clearly the preferred option. Here's how it might sound with a teacher giving it a try: "Jose, I've noticed that it is very hard for you to settle down to work when you come in from the hallway for science. But when you have difficulty settling down it makes it hard for the other kids to get their work done and then I have to get on your case. Can we think about how we can help you settle down without me having to get on your case?"

Now, how might continuous practice at (preferably Proactive) Plan B help a child shift set more readily? Children and adults who shift cognitive set rapidly and efficiently tend to rely heavily on their ability to anticipate the need to shift before the environment demands the shift. Such anticipation engenders advance preparation for finishing one thing and moving to another, and therefore reduces the likelihood of surprises. Children and adults who have difficulty shifting cognitive set often have a limited capacity for such anticipation, and therefore experience a lot of surprises (along wth the arousal and affect that typically accompany surprises). Proactive Plan B helps children and adults anticipate routine shifts and prepare in advance. Such practice may also (eventually) help the child deal more effectively with shifts that are not routine. Further, solving problems collaboratively helps the child actively contemplate how to navigate shifts rather than simply being on the receiving end of a demand to shift. As with other skills trained with Proactive Plan B, it is likely that the child will require some "in-the-moment" training as well.

Language-Processing Skills

Several skills related to the language pathway were also discussed in the first section of this chapter. However, we've yet to discuss how to train a basic vocabulary for expressing and categorizing emotions, which will require some modification to basic Plan B. Many children who lack such a vocabulary express their frustration through profanity. While we've seen swearing set in motion vigorous attempts to teach the child "respect for authority," we find that teaching a more adaptive vocabulary for articulating emotions is likely to be a more productive pursuit. Regardless of age, we like to keep it simple and start with a rudimentary vocabulary such as *happy, sad, frustrated*, and *nervous* or *worried*. Here's what the initial Proactive Plan B discussion might sound like when aimed at helping the child to develop this basic feeling vocabulary. While this discussion could take place in a therapy session, let's assume the surrogate frontal lobe was able to go it alone:

ADULT: (*empathy*) I've noticed that sometimes you get very upset about things around here.

CHILD: Yeah.

ADULT: (*defining the problem*) I'm not mad about it, but I sure would like to see if we could give you words to use to tell me you're upset besides the one's you've been using.

CHILD: Yeah.

ADULT: (*reassurance and invitation*) I'm not saying you can't get upset . . . but I wonder if we could think of something you could say when you're frustrated besides "Screw you"?

CHILD: Not really.

ADULT: I have some ideas . . . would you like to hear them?

CHILD: OK.

ADULT: How about "I'm frustrated"?

Of course, as with the vocabularies being trained in the first section of

this chapter, there will be probably be a need for some "in-the-moment" reminders of this new vocabulary at times when the child is clearly at, shall we
say, a loss for (appropriate) words. So when a child screams "Screw you!," it is
the job of the surrogate frontal lobe to kick in with the vocabulary: "Boy, you're
frustrated!" Over time—after many repetitions—we find that children and
adolescents begin to utilize their new vocabulary. This does not happen immediately, of course, and the clinician must remind the adults that remediating
learning disabilities can take a while. But if a lack of a feeling vocabulary is the
problem we're trying to fix, we know of no faster way to get the job done. It is
also worth reminding adults that since thousands of prior Plan A repetitions
have yet to fix the problem, they have little to lose by throwing their fates to
the Plan B winds.

Is it hard for adults to react to inappropriate language in such a way? Yes,
absolutely. Indeed, most adults find it difficult to resist the temptation to remind the child that he is not supposed to talk that way before getting around to
training the new vocabulary. While we understand this instinct, we also find
that the child already knows that profanity is inappropriate (having been told
so many times before). Further, providing a more adaptive vocabulary ("You're
frustrated") sends the very message that the words the child used were less
than adaptive but without running the risk of escalating the child with Plan A
and rendering him a less available learner. Thus, it's also important to remind
adults that they are "setting limits" whether they're using Plan A or Plan B, especially when one understands that "limit setting" is defined as *ensuring that
an adult's concerns are addressed.*

By the way, one of the reasons we've devoted an entire chapter in this
book to implementation of CPS in school settings (Chapter 7) is because we
are aware that the preceding paragraph (perhaps many other paragraphs as
well!) will be met with understandable skepticism by adults trying to intervene in the company of 25–30 students in a classroom. Indeed, the natural instinct when a student says "Screw you!" in a classroom setting (often mandated by the school discipline code) is to demand that the child immediately
leave the setting, in favor of a seat in the hallway or to one in the assistant principal's office. It's worth pointing out that neither of these seats trains a new
feeling vocabulary and therefore doesn't fix the problem. And if a teacher is
understandably concerned that a Plan B dialogue in response to "Screw you!"
will interrupt the learning of other students, we would suggest that the 2–3
minutes spent modeling a new skill or solving a problem collaboratively may
be the most important teaching that takes place in the classroom the entire
school day . . . even for the students who don't have apparent difficulties with
the skill or problem solving.

It can also be useful to provide the child with opportunities to practice his new feeling vocabulary once it has been introduced. For instance, this might take the form of brief (daily) discussions about the new vocabulary outside the heat of the moment. At home such discussions can take place at bedtime or when driving in the car. At school, such discussions can take place whenever the adult can grab an opportune moment to have a brief, one-on-one discussion with a student. The purpose of these discussions is simply to review various situations and support the new feeling vocabulary. Here's how one such discussion might sound: "Remember this morning when your brother spilled his drink on your homework? How did that make you feel?" (In initial discussions, the child is likely to respond with "I don't know.") "I think you were probably frustrated. Your face looked frustrated . . . it's something people would usually get frustrated about . . . I think frustrated is what you were." Likewise, adults can help children observe and label the emotional states of others throughout the day. Books, stories, picture cards, TV cartoons, and billboards offer nice opportunities for practicing a new feeling vocabulary. We find that this additional practice with the new vocabulary under optimal circumstances can speed skill acquisition.

Emotion Regulation Skills

As we discussed in Chapter 1, difficulties with emotion regulation can be either acute (a skill we've referred to as separation of affect) or more pervasive. Regarding the former, recall that separation of affect requires that a person suspend his or her emotional reaction to a particular problem or disagreement in order to think clearly about potential response options. We've found that basic Plan B can be effective at teaching this skill. Empathy is, of course, crucial to this process, for it ensures that the child's concern is not only understood, acknowledged, and validated but also considered first. Thus, much of the emotional arousal produced by Plan A—in which the adult's concern is not only the first but also the only concern entered into consideration—is diminished. In our experience, few kids react in a highly emotional way to empathy (unless, for example, they have learned that empathy is merely a segue into Plan A). Some children can have a strong reaction to the second step of Plan B (problem definition), but many such children become less aroused with a dose of reassurance (once again, being assured that consideration of an adult concern does not portend the arrival of Plan A). Over time—as the child learns that solutions to problems actually do take his concerns into account—reactivity to problems and frustrations is further reduced.

While many kids with more chronic or pervasive irritability and/or anxiety may ultimately require pharmacological intervention—as noted earlier, these are difficulties medication is often effective at treating—we do not automatically think of medication when these difficulties are present. Indeed, there is a growing literature suggesting that cognitive interventions for depression and anxiety in children and adolescents can actually be quite effective. Our goal here is not to present a review of this literature, but rather to focus on the mechanism by which the problem solving that takes place with basic Plan B can serve to reduce anxiety and irritability. Proactive Plan B can be useful for the purpose of helping children recognize situations that routinely result in anxiety or irritability:

PARENT: Sara, I've noticed that you've been in a very bad mood lately whenever you get home from a visit at your father's.

ADOLESCENT: How can you tell?

PARENT: Well, you're usually a pretty happy kid, but when you get home from your father's you've been kind of cranky and grumpy.

ADOLESCENT: How can you tell I'm cranky and grumpy?

PARENT: Well, you get very quiet . . . you sigh a lot . . . sometimes you blow up at me . . . that's not like you.

After numerous repetitions of this sort of dialogue, we would expect that a child would be able to recognize and articulate a mood state without need of prompting. Of course, the conversation would continue to determine the nature of the problem and generate potential mutually satisfactory solutions:

PARENT: What's up? Anything I can help with?

ADOLESCENT: You guys want me to be happy even though you're divorced, but I'm not.

PARENT: I hear you. I know you're not happy about it. It is hard.

ADOLESCENT: Well, that's it . . . there's nothing anyone can do about it.

PARENT: I don't know about that.

ADOLESCENT: Well, you're not getting back together, are you?

PARENT: No, I don't think that's going to happen. But I wonder if there's anything we can do to help you be happier even though we're not going to get back together. I guess I need a better idea of what it is about us being divorced that is making you so unhappy. Is it that we're not all together as a family anymore . . . or that it's a hassle to move from one house to another?

Moreover, we've worked with many children and adolescents whose irritability and anxieties could be traced back to *chronic problems that were perpetually unsolved*.

THERAPIST: (*empathy*) Kevin, I understand you've been skipping school.

KEVIN: I hate that freaking place.

THERAPIST: How come you're skipping school?

KEVIN: I don't know.

THERAPIST: When did you first start skipping school?

KEVIN: A few years ago.

THERAPIST: Why did you start skipping school back then?

KEVIN: I couldn't keep up in my classes, and no one was giving me any help, so I just blew it off.

THERAPIST: (*empathy*) Do you think that's why you're skipping school now? You're so far behind, it feels like it would be impossible to catch up?

KEVIN: Yeah. I mean, what's the point?

THERAPIST: (*defining the problem*) Of course, if you keep skipping, you'll have absolutely no chance of catching up. Plus, you get into trouble.

KEVIN: It doesn't matter. I don't care anymore.

THERAPIST: I can understand how you got to that point. But I'm just wondering if there's anything we could do to get things back on track.

Now, as we have noted elsewhere, a child with explosive outbursts does not automatically qualify as having difficulties with emotion regulation. Along these lines, we should add a note of concern here about the alarming rates at which bipolar disorder in particular is being diagnosed in children and our equal concern about the high rates at which atypical antipsychotic medication and other mood stabilizers are being prescribed. We do not question the legitimacy of the bipolar disorder diagnosis in children, but we do question the prevalence rates offered by some research labs and the manner by which adult criteria for mania have been adjusted to fit children. Our experience is that many children are being diagnosed with bipolar disorder without a comprehensive evaluation and without consideration of the cognitive and situational factors that may also contribute to explosiveness, oppositionality, hyperactivity, and irritability.

Thus, while we also do not question the potential effectiveness of atypical antipsychotics and other mood-stabilizing medications—for we have certainly seen such medications produce extraordinary improvements in many children (and an emerging research literature has begun to confirm this anecdotal impression)—we do question the frequency by which the bipolar diagnosis is being made in the absence of any recognized or universally sanctioned criteria, and the apparent ease with which many practitioners have placed children who are so diagnosed on a potent class of medication.

There are many reasons why a child might react poorly to frustration (the emotional reactivity of bipolar disorder being but one). Our sense is that the diagnosis of juvenile bipolar disorder has, in many children, essentially become a proxy for the combination of severe oppositionality, irritability, and hyperactivity.

As you might imagine, our biggest concern with the diagnosis of bipolar disorder in children is that, like other diagnoses, it does not help us understand the cognitive factors underlying the child's difficulties. We believe this is the danger whenever diagnoses—rather than etiological models and conceptualizations of underlying pathogenic mechanisms—guide treatment selection. Indeed, the diagnosis of pediatric bipolar disorder leads to an almost instantaneous assumption of neurobiochemical underpinnings (and therefore instantaneous consideration of medical intervention). The reality is that mood stabilizers do not, and cannot be expected to, address the myriad cognitive issues we see in many of the children who carry the diagnosis. See McClellan (2005) for further discussion of these issues.

Cognitive Flexibility Skills

Recall that children whose lagging cognitive skills are found in the cognitive flexibility category typically approach the world in a very black-and-white, literal, rigid manner. These are children who tend to be strong at memorizing factual information and deal well with the world when life is predictable, but have difficulties with "grayer" aspects of living, such as problem solving, social interactions, and unpredictable circumstances. One well-known by-product of this cognitive profile is anxiety, for these children are uncomfortable in situations in which they have no frame of reference or have little sense of mastery. Less documented is the poor tolerance for frustration (and resulting explosive outbursts) that can be a by-product of the child's discomfort in novel situations or circumstances demanding a flexible approach to problem solving and social interactions. As social skills are discussed below, we shall focus in this section on the manner by which Plan B would address some of the unique problem-solving difficulties of children with this profile.

The calming component of the first step of Plan B (empathy/reassurance) is crucial for such children, as they often overreact when faced with the realization that their rigid notions about how events should unfold will not be fulfilled. Moreover, we find that, because their rigid concerns can seem quite unreasonable to the untrained listener, these children have grown accustomed to having adults (and often peers as well) instantaneously reject their ideas. No matter how far-fetched their concerns may be, as with any child prone to explosive episodes, we find it immensely helpful to make sure that their concerns are acknowledged. So the fact that empathy ensures that the child's concern is entered into consideration is crucial.

We find that "cognitively inflexible" children often define problems in a very rigid manner. Indeed, because of their difficulties with perspective taking, they may have extreme difficulty taking another person's concerns into account. The second step of Plan B (problem definition) provides the child with a mechanism for considering another person's concern and sets the parameters for solving the problem. Remember, the child doesn't have to "own" your concern to assist in solving the problem; he merely needs to take it into account in working toward a mutually satisfactory solution. Sometimes, helping a rigid, inflexible child simply *hear* someone else's concern is a major therapeutic achievement. This is often accomplished by stating the adult concern in a more tentative or nuanced fashion than might ordinarily be the case. In other words, if the child is a black-and-white thinker who says "black," then the surrogate frontal lobe first needs to acknowledge "black" and, rather than saying anything that sounds too close to "white," instead insert something that is a few shades "grayer" than "black"!

MOTHER: It's supposed to snow later today and I just know that Hannah is going to lose it if her gymnastics class is canceled. Plus she's decided that since it's almost spring there won't be any more snow!

THERAPIST: Well, sounds like the time to start working on that problem is right now—before it comes up.

MOTHER: I'm afraid to even bring it up. I have no idea how to do it.

THERAPIST: Let's bring Hannah in and see if we can do it together. It's a nice opportunity to practice Proactive Plan B.

(*Hannah joins her mother, father, and therapist in the room.*)

MOTHER: Hannah, I heard on the news before we came over here that it's probably going to snow today. And I was thinking that . . .

HANNAH: It is not! Look outside! It's not even snowing! Besides, spring starts on Saturday, so it can't!

MOTHER: (*Looks to therapist, feeling lost.*)

THERAPIST: Hannah, are you worried that gymnastics will get canceled today because of the snow?

HANNAH: It's not going to snow!

THERAPIST: (*acknowledging Hannah's rigid idea and beginning to nuance, but without arguing*) You know you might be right. It might not snow at all today or anymore this year even! [Notice the word "might" instead of the word "won't."]

HANNAH: Good!

THERAPIST: (*searching for the gray shades that exist between black and white*) Has it ever snowed when you didn't think it would?

HANNAH: Nope. Never.

THERAPIST: (*doesn't argue*) Wow! You're good at predicting it then, huh? I'm pretty good at knowing when it's going to snow, too. Of course, sometimes the snow surprises me.

HANNAH: Well, it doesn't surprise me. The weatherman on TV said that spring starts this Saturday.

THERAPIST: Yes, I heard that spring starts this Saturday. I can't wait to start planting my garden. Of course, there was that one year that I didn't think it was going to snow again so I planted my garden and then the snow surprised me.

HANNAH: It did? What did you do?

THERAPIST: I had to replant a bunch of stuff. I was pretty upset about that. [Having now helped Sarah begin to consider the possibility of surprise snow, the therapist feels safer moving on to a more refined definition of the problem.] Tell me, besides that it's almost spring, how come you don't want it to snow?

HANNAH: I hate when my stuff gets canceled.

THERAPIST: Like gymnastics?

HANNAH: Yes. I have it today. That's why it's not going to be canceled.

THERAPIST: Yes, if it doesn't snow, gymnastics won't get canceled. I hope the snow doesn't surprise us!

HANNAH: Me too!

THERAPIST: What will happen if the snow does surprise you? You know, like it once surprised me with my garden? What will you do if gymnastics gets canceled?

HANNAH: I don't know!

THERAPIST: Should we think about some things you can do if gymnastics gets canceled by surprise snow?

HANNAH: I don't know. This is boring. I don't want to talk about this anymore!

MOTHER: We have to, honey, so we can figure out how to fix things like this so you don't get all upset.

HANNAH: I don't want to!

THERAPIST: [Having made good headway in one Plan B conversation, the therapist is concerned about diminishing returns.] Let's stop talking about it then. Hannah, why don't you go back out to the waiting room and your parents will be out in just a minute. You did a good job of talking with us. (*turns to parents after Hannah has left*) The problem isn't solved yet. But she was able to hang with the discussion and contemplate that the snow might surprise her and even talk about why that is upsetting to her. That's progress. The next step is for her to tolerate talking about how to solve the problem. Slow work, but we're getting there.

MOTHER: Is she ever going to be able to do this?

THERAPIST: Well, we haven't been at it for very long. And I think she is doing it. She's just not all the way there yet. But I'm not seeing anything that makes me feel like she won't be able to begin contemplating solutions pretty soon. I think it's a big step just for her to hang in there with our attempts to slightly modify her existing ways of thinking.

It was important to end the session by underscoring the progress that was being made even though the ultimate goal had yet to be achieved. It was also important to remind the adults that teaching a rigid thinker to approach problems in more flexible ways requires practice. For this reason, often the first goal is not to arrive at wonderful, mutually satisfactory solutions to problems but rather to have the child tolerate the idea that there might be some shades of gray somewhere between black and white.

Along these lines, an attempted Plan B conversation hasn't "failed" because the participants didn't make it through all three steps on the first try. If an attempted Plan B discussion has set the stage for later resumption, we'd consider the attempt a success. Some children often have very limited problem-solving repertoires: "This is the way it has to be! There is no other way!" In combination with massive doses of empathy, the third step of Plan B (the invitation) sets the stage for these children to access the full range of possibilities for solving a problem, to remain cognizant of the fact that their concerns will be taken into account, and to achieve a comfort level with brainstorming. We find that such children often benefit from being reminded about how they have resolved similar problems in the past so that they might more readily see the connection between past solutions and current problems.

Here's an example of a teacher attempting such training using Proactive Plan B:

TEACHER: Evan, we have a bit of a problem with recess tomorrow.

EVAN: What do you mean?

TEACHER: Well, we have an assembly tomorrow during recess, so I thought we could talk about that today before it happens.

EVAN: Why are we talking about it now?

TEACHER: I remember that the last time we didn't go out for recess at the usual time it was very upsetting to you.

EVAN: It's not a problem right now.

TEACHER: Well, I know that, but come tomorrow it's likely to be a problem.

EVAN: So what? I'm not going to talk about a problem that isn't a problem yet. I mean you can't have a problem before it's a problem. There is no problem right now, so there's nothing to talk about.

TEACHER: OK. Gotcha. You're right. There is no problem right now. That is 100% correct. I'm just thinking that if we spend a few minutes on it now, then you we won't have to deal with it tomorrow.

EVAN: But how can we talk about a problem that is not even a problem!?

TEACHER: You're right. We can't. So let's just spend 5 minutes talking about pretend problems since problems can't exist unless they're already problems. [Notice how the teacher empathizes with Evan's rigid and literal stance without trying to convince Evan that it is incorrect.]

EVAN: OK.

TEACHER: Let's just pretend that it's tomorrow and there's an assembly during recess.

EVAN: What time's the assembly?

TEACHER: 10:15.

EVAN: There can't be an assembly at 10:15 . . . we have recess at 10:15.

TEACHER: Yes, that's the problem

EVAN: It's not a problem for me. I'm going out for recess at 10:15.

TEACHER: Well, that's an option, I suppose. The only problem is, there won't be anyone else at recess except you. [Remember, there's no such thing as a bad idea. The teacher's role here is to test out possible solutions.]

EVAN: I don't care. I'm going out for recess at 10:15.

TEACHER: You know what I'm thinking? I'm thinking this problem has come up before. There was another time we couldn't go to recess when we were supposed to . . .

EVAN: It wasn't the same thing.

TEACHER: It wasn't? I don't remember what it was the last time, do you?

EVAN: That time it was a fire drill that kept us from going out for recess at 10:15.

TEACHER: Oh, right. So that wasn't the same thing.

EVAN: Right. It's not the same thing.

TEACHER: I was just thinking that the solution that worked the last time might work this time . . . even though it's not the exact same thing. When it was the fire drill we went out for recess at 11:15 instead.

EVAN: Right.

TEACHER: Do you think that could work this time . . . even though it's not the exact same thing? That way, you'd have all your friends at recess with you instead of being out there all alone. What do you think?

EVAN: I wish recess was at 10:15.

TEACHER: Me, too. I don't like it when they change the schedule. But do you think 11:15 would work? It worked the last time.

EVAN: Is recess at 10:15 the next day?

TEACHER: Yes, it is.

EVAN: OK.

TEACHER: Thanks for helping me figure this out, buddy.

EVAN: OK.

Here's another example along the same lines:

MOTHER: Last night was not a good night.

THERAPIST: How come?

MOTHER: We had a pretty big blowup around bedtime.

THERAPIST: JD, do you want to tell me what happened?

JD: My brother was in the bathroom! That's what!

THERAPIST: OK. Your brother was in the bathroom. Tell me why that was a problem. I'm assuming it was because you wanted to be in there?

MOTHER: Well, his bathroom routine got disrupted and so his father tried to help him to do things in our bathroom instead, but let's just say it backfired.

JD: That's not my routine! I told them that!

THERAPIST: That's not your routine. Tell me what your routine is.

JD: I brush my teeth, use my fluoride rinse, make a pee, and then go into my bedroom to get my pajamas on.

THERAPIST: And you couldn't do that because your brother was in there first?

MOTHER: His brother takes a while to go to the bathroom (*laughing*).

THERAPIST: OK. Gotcha. So, JD, you were ready to do your routine and your brother sort of messed it up—even though he was just trying to go to the bathroom.

JD: Right!

MOTHER: So his father brought JD's pajamas into our bathroom so he could change there and do the rest of the things.

JD: But I don't put my pajamas on in the bathroom! And you don't have the fluoride rinse in your bathroom anyway!

MOTHER: I know, honey, but Daddy was just trying to help and sometimes you need to be a little flexible.

THERAPIST: One thing we know about JD is that he likes to have a routine that he can depend on.

MOTHER: But you can't always have the same routine! Sometimes things happen and you need to be flexible.

THERAPIST: That's absolutely true, and I don't think the problem is that JD *won't* deviate from a routine—I just think he needs to have a plan for figuring out what that different way would be. JD, you like Rescue Heroes, right?

JD: Yup.

THERAPIST: When the Rescue Heroes go to perform a rescue, do they have a plan?

JD: Of course.

THERAPIST: And what if something goes wrong and that plan won't work for some reason?

JD: Then they go to Plan B!

THERAPIST: Plan B! You mean they have more than one plan?

JD: You always have to have a backup plan.

THERAPIST: So maybe what we need here—for when the usual plan doesn't work—is a backup plan. Like with the nighttime routine, there was a problem with the usual plan, yes?

JD: Yes!

THERAPIST: Because your brother was in the bathroom?

JD: Right! We needed a Plan B!

THERAPIST: What might Plan B have looked like?

JD: Well, I could have used my parents' bathroom but then gone back into my room for pajamas.

MOTHER: But you just said that we don't have your toothbrush and the rinse in there.

JD: You could bring it in if we're doing Plan B.

THERAPIST: Mom, does that work for you?

MOTHER: Sure. I don't have a problem with that. It's not much different than what we actually suggested last night, though.

JD: Yes it is.

MOTHER: Why, aside from the pajamas?

JD: Because you didn't let me help with the new plan.

When adults use Plan A to solve problems, the child has no ownership of the solution. We find that children—like other members of the human species—are much more receptive to discussing solutions that haven't panned out when they have participated in the creation of the solution than when adults impose solutions. We also think that discussing problems in a manner that enhances adult–child communication is far more effective than handling problems in a way (Plan A) that *reduces* the likelihood of future communication.

As we noted in Chapter 1, black-and-white thinking can also set the stage for biased, inflexible interpretations of one's experiences, such as "I'm stu-pid," "It's not fair," "You always blame me," "People are out to get me," "You can't trust adults," and "Nobody likes me." Consistent with Aaron Beck's work in identifying errors in logic in adults (e.g., overgeneralization, catastrophizing, personalization), Plan B can be used to help children think and interpret their experiences in more realistic and adaptive ways. The goals for the surrogate frontal lobe are to identify cognitive biases or distortions and to provide disconfirming evidence at opportune moments. As always, these goals are more easily accomplished through use of Proactive B than Emergency B.

In the following example, a teacher is working with a third-grade girl to help her first recognize a cognitive distortion and then to help her move to-ward a more accurate, flexible interpretation of her experience by providing disconfirming evidence at key opportunities.

TEACHER: *(empathy, using Proactive B)* I hear you saying you're stupid sometimes. What's up?

CHILD: I'm stupid!

TEACHER: *(attempting to clarify)* Yes, I heard you say so.

CHILD: So you think I'm stupid, too!

TEACHER: No, I actually don't, but I was just wondering why you think you're stupid.

CHILD: I stink in reading!

TEACHER: *(re-empathizing, now that the child's concern has been clarified)* Ah, so you think you're stupid because you have some trouble in read-ing.

CHILD: Yes, I'm in that stupid reading group.

TEACHER: *(defining the problem)* Yes, you are in the group of kids who need some extra help in reading. I'm just not sure if that makes you stupid. You're very good in math—in fact, you help a lot of the other kids in math—so it's hard for me to think of you as stupid.

CHILD: Well, I *am* stupid!

TEACHER: *(inviting)* I wonder if there's some other way to think about read-ing being a little hard for you besides that you're stupid. Do you have any ideas?

CHILD: Like what?

TEACHER: Well, like maybe that you're really good in math but still need some extra help in reading.

On numerous subsequent occasions, when the teacher was handing math quizzes back to her students, she would provide disconfirming evidence and remind the girl of the alternative interpretation by going over to the girl and whispering in her ear, "I know you sometimes say you're stupid but you got the highest grade in the class on the math quiz again. Looks to me like you're really good in math but still need some extra help in reading." It took a while, but three months later the girl was heard proudly announcing to her peers on the playground, "Oh, I'm good in math, but I just need some extra help in reading."

These principles can be applied to a wide range of cognitive distortions, so long as the adult realizes that most distortions have some basis in reality. So empathy—letting the child know that her concern (in this case, her belief) is heard and taken seriously—is crucial, even as the adult encourages more flexible and accurate beliefs.

Social Skills

You may recall from Chapter 1 that the outbursts of many explosive kids are often attributable to difficulties in social skills, including failing to understand how one's behavior is affecting other people, failing to take another person's perspective into account, having a narrow repertoire of social responses, failing to appreciate (often nonverbal) social nuances, failing to recognize how one's behavior is being perceived by others, and pragmatic issues (starting a conversation, entering a group, etc.). Some of these skills, by the way, are trained simply by using Plan B (e.g., at a very basic level, one must take another's perspective into account to generate and agree upon mutually satisfactory solutions). Others must be trained more directly. The social skills training literature is expansive, and it is not feasible to provide here a review of the many different strategies for training these additional skills. Rather, our goal is to provide a few examples of how the training of these skills might be facilitated with Plan B. Our focus in this section is on cognitive deficiencies, as we discussed cognitive distortions in the emotion regulation section of this chapter.

We should point out that one advantage of Plan B is that it sets the stage for training to occur *in the environments in which the skills are to be utilized*. We think this has major ramifications for maintenance of the trained skills. Most cognitive skills training programs are designed to provide training *outside* the environments in which the skills are actually to be performed . . . in other words, in a guidance counselor's office, a therapist's office, or a researcher's lab. We believe this may at least partially explain why the skills training literature reveals serious problems with maintenance and generalization of treatment effects. When people who interact with a child in the real world are training and helping the child practice the skills, concerns about maintenance and generalization tend to fade.

Another advantage of Plan B, as it relates to teaching social skills, is that it is *collaborative*. Thus, there's a better chance that the child will actually *think about* a given problem or issue and contemplate potential solutions. Again, such a process lends itself to greater ownership of both the problem and the solutions. In many social skills training programs, information regarding adaptive social functioning is taught in a more didactic fashion. And with Plan A, of course, the child is simply told what to do differently ("You need to share or I'm taking the toys away"). By contrast, here's how an adult might attempt a Proactive Plan B discussion with an adolescent having difficulty, for example, appreciating the impact of his behavior on others:

ADULT: (*empathy*) Marvin, I know you like kidding around with your younger sister.

MARVIN: Yeah?

ADULT: And I know your sister loves hanging around with you.

MARVIN: (*a little agitated*) Is there a point here?

ADULT: (*define the problem*) Well, my concern is that some of your kidding is making your sister feel bad.

MARVIN: (*a little more agitated*) What are you talking about?

ADULT: Well, I don't think she thinks it's funny when you call her "Sisterwife."

MARVIN: She does think it's funny!

ADULT: I know you *think* she does, but she's come to me several times to tell me it bothers her. She also doesn't think it's funny when you hump the couch in front of her.

MARVIN: I don't do that!

ADULT: Um, I've seen you do it a few times.

MARVIN: What is the point of this conversation?

ADULT: Well, I think sometimes you're not aware that some of the things you do are troubling to other people.

MARVIN: What are you, my shrink? This is pissing me off!

ADULT: (*invitation*) I don't mean to piss you off. We don't have to talk about it right now. But I was wondering if we could do something about the problem.

MARVIN: It's not a problem!

ADULT: It is for your sister. It makes her very uncomfortable.

MARVIN: Fine, I won't do it anymore!

ADULT: Do you understand why it makes her uncomfortable?

MARVIN: I don't care! I said I'd stop!

ADULT: I appreciate that. Do you understand?

MARVIN: Yes! Leave me alone!

ADULT: Let's see how things go . . . maybe we'll talk about this again.

MARVIN: I'm not talking about it again!

If it seems that this brief discussion is unlikely to accomplish the mission, you're right. Hopefully, the adult understands that this is only the beginning of what could be an ongoing dialogue on the topic. Rome wasn't built in a day. This conversation just gets the Plan B ball rolling. Marvin might be a bit more receptive if it turns out that his solution ("Fine, I won't do it anymore!") doesn't quite get the job done, especially if an adult points this out to him by offering additional help rather than by issuing a demand or an admonition.

Here's another example of how Proactive Plan B can be used to teach pragmatic social skills:

GREG: My life sucks.

THERAPIST: (*basic empathy*) Your life sucks? How so?

GREG: I never do anything fun. All I do is sit home and play video games.

THERAPIST: How come you don't do more things with your friends from school?

GREG: Well, I do stuff with them, but only if they ask me to do something. But I never ask them to do stuff.

THERAPIST: How come?

GREG: I don't know how to, so I just don't.

THERAPIST: (*refined empathy, then invitation*) You don't know how to ask people to do something outside school, so you end up spending more time by yourself—which can get pretty lonely. Any ideas how this problem could get solved?

GREG: Well, it's not just that I don't know how to ask people. If I get together with someone I'm not sure what to do—like if it's not planned for us. You know in school you don't have to think about what you are going to do. But like if someone comes over to my house I don't know what we would do.

THERAPIST: Sounds like we also need to figure out how to help you plan things so you feel comfortable knowing what you'll be doing. Yes?

GREG: Yes.

THERAPIST: So let's think of a plan.

GREG: Well, Jason likes the movies. We could go to a movie—so then we wouldn't have to talk!

THERAPIST: That's an idea . . .

GREG: But I don't know what we would talk about on the way there . . . or after the movie.

THERAPIST: First of all, it's OK not to talk the whole time you're with someone. Sometimes there's nothing to say. But what do people talk about in casual conversations with each other?

GREG: I don't know.

THERAPIST: Let's think about it. I think two general topics are things that are going on in their lives and things they have in common . . . you know, common interests.

GREG: Hmm.

THERAPIST: Do you and Jason have some things in common that you might be able to talk about easily?

GREG: Um . . . yeah . . . I think so.

THERAPIST: OK. Like what?

GREG: Video games. And movies. But that's at school.

THERAPIST: Any reason you guys couldn't talk about that stuff on the way to the movies?

GREG: Um . . . I guess not.

THERAPIST: OK, so how do you feel about the movies as the activity?

GREG: Good.

THERAPIST: Do you feel like you have a pretty good idea of things you could talk about before and after the movie?

GREG: Yes. I think so.

THERAPIST: Should we talk about the words you could use to invite Jason to the movies?

GREG: OK.

Naturally, the discussion would continue until all of Greg's concerns were addressed and a definitive plan arrived upon. Of course, the larger problem is not yet solved . . . Greg's social difficulties will require ongoing problem solving and planning.

Q & A

I understand that certain skills are necessary for a child or adult to participate in Plan B and that these skills might need to be trained. But in Chapter 4, you distinguished between "problem-focused Plan B" and "skill-focused Plan B," and I'd like to hear a little more about that.

At any point in treatment—but hopefully early on—it may become apparent that a specific problem or trigger (e.g., doing homework, eating healthy foods, taking medicine, getting to bed at night, waking up in the morning) is precipitating a large number of explosive episodes. *Problem-focused Plan B* refers to any Plan B discussion aimed at resolving such problems or triggers. In other instances, it may be apparent that a specific lagging thinking skill—for example, difficulty appreciating the impact of one's behavior on others, black-and-white thinking, difficulty shifting cognitive set, difficulty putting one's thoughts into words—is setting the stage for explosive episodes cutting across multiple situations. *Skill-focused Plan B* refers to any Plan B discussion aimed at teaching these skills.

For example, if a child balks at turning off the television to come in for dinner, and this scenario causes a meaningful number of explosive episodes, a problem-focused Plan B discussion would center on resolving that particular problem. So if the child's concern is that his favorite show is being interrupted and the adult's concern is that it's important to eat together as a family, then the two parties should try to arrive at a solution that would address these concerns. But if it becomes apparent that the child has difficulty shifting from one activity to another across multiple circumstances (e.g., going to school, going to bed at night, coming indoors after playing outside), then skill-focused Plan B (aimed at enhancing the general skill of shifting cognitive set) might well be more productive. In such cases, the focus of Plan B shifts from a specific problem (TV show being interrupted/eating dinner together) to the training of a specific skill (shifting cognitive set). Indeed, in many cases where problem-focused Plan B is the initial approach for addressing a given cluster of explosive episodes, it becomes evident that a specific lagging skill is coming into play and that a more productive approach would be to focus directly on teaching the specific skill (skill-focused Plan B), at least for that cluster of explosive episodes.

Deciding whether to emphasize problem-focused Plan B or skill-focused Plan B is completely a matter of clinical judgment and may involve consideration of other factors such as a child's level of stability (sometimes addressing a particularly problematic trigger can have a dramatic stabilizing effect) or the degree to which caretakers fully understand the specific lagging skills underlying a child's challenges and how these skills can be trained (sometimes, especially early in treatment, problem-focused Plan B is easier for caretakers to understand and implement).

You've also mentioned that Plan B can be useful as an assessment tool. I'd like to hear more about that, too.

As you know, the first step of Plan B (empathy) is aimed at ensuring that a child's concern is well understood and being entered into consideration. Crucial assessment information can be gathered in attempting to clarify a child's concern.

Let's use the example of a resident in a therapeutic facility balking at attending group therapy. A staff member might initiate a Proactive Plan B discussion as follows: "I've noticed that you haven't been too enthusiastic about going to group therapy lately. What's up?" The resident's response should provide important assessment information (and also inform whether the ensuing discussion is problem-focused or skill-focused). For example, if the resident responds, "You know Billy has bad body odor—I just can't stand sitting in the same room with him," then problem-focused Plan B will likely ensue. But if the resident responds, "Everyone wants me to say stuff in there .. . they want me to talk .. . and I don't know what to say," we might want to explore further some of the specific items contained within the language-processing pathway. Or if the resident responds, "Look, man, all people do in there is talk about their problems .. . I'm feeling bad enough about my life without getting dragged down by other people's problems," further inquiry might well focus on items within the emotion regulation pathway.

Can Plan B be effective in dealing with sibling interactions?

Absolutely, but we usually wait until adult caretakers have mastered Plan B in their own interactions with their explosive child before extending their role to what is usually a more difficult circumstance: facilitating a Plan

B discussion between siblings. Much of the discussion about student–student interactions in Chapter 7 is also applicable to sibling interactions.

How long does treatment typically last?

Although managed care dictates the answer to this question to some degree, the preferred answer is "as long as necessary." Not unlike other treatment modalities, however, treatment duration is highly variable. Our research suggests that 80% of parents report significant reductions in explosive behavior after 10 or fewer sessions. Many parents require only a session or two. Many other parents—especially those who have significant lagging skills of their own, and/or children who are at the more severe end of the explosiveness spectrum—require more time. And some parents continue to need our assistance, at least on an intermittent basis, for longer periods.

What if a child refuses to come to therapy?

As depicted in the dialogue earlier in this chapter, we assume he has a good reason for it. We don't think it's strategically wise to force a child to come to therapy, so coming to therapy is not handled with Plan A. We have sent parents home from therapy with the assignment of telling the child that we want to hear their side of the story or that we want to know more about what the parents are doing wrong. This isn't a trick . . . we actually do want to know.

I have many additional questions!

Outstanding. Many of the additional questions clinicians have about the CPS model are answered in Chapter 9. In the next two chapters, we turn our attention to implementation of the model in larger systems.

Chapter 7

Collaborative Problem
Solving in Schools

Schools present many significant challenges to implementation of the CPS model. At the same time, CPS has the potential to benefit students and teachers substantially. Obviously, the model can significantly influence one-on-one teacher–student interactions, and the information presented in the previous chapters is, of course, relevant along these lines. But CPS is also applicable to other types of interactions in schools, such as child–child interactions (i.e., between classmates) and adult–adult interactions (e.g., interactions among teachers, between teachers and administrators, and between teachers and parents). In addition, there are a variety of additional challenges that come into play when applying the CPS model in larger groups and in systems.

By far the biggest challenge to the implementation of CPS in schools is *inertia*: many people find it difficult to change course when they have been doing something a certain way for a long time. School discipline programs have historically relied heavily on reward-and-punishment procedures, often without anyone having taken notice of the fact that the students who are the most frequent recipients of "discipline" (often in the form of detention, suspension, expulsion, and, in the "good old days," paddling) are those who derive the least benefit from these interventions (see the excellent work of Mark Atkins and

154

colleagues [Atkins et al., 2002]). Changing the direction of the rusting hulk of a ship called the "school discipline program" takes a great deal of time and perseverance. The simplicity and systematic nature of the CPS model can mitigate the inertia. Indeed, at a very basic level, CPS requires that adults merely have an understanding of *five pathways, three plans, and three steps for doing Plan B.*

By the way, it is not uncommon for school personnel to expect parents to rectify the explosive behavior of their children at school. As the parents generally aren't even present when explosive episodes occur at school, they are unlikely to be the most important players as it relates to resolving behavior problems at school (although they are likely to be very important collaborators).

A second major challenge is the lack of a *philosophy* . . . about children in general and about why children behave in a maladaptive fashion in particular. Philosophy is important because it guides our actions, especially when the going gets rough. If a school system or a particular school or teacher has no philosophy, responses to explosive kids depend more on the prevailing winds, on existing but frequently ineffective disciplinary programs, or on what works best for the larger group. As you know, the CPS model conceives of challenging behavior as the byproduct of lagging cognitive skills, and the philosophy of the model—*"Children do well if they can"*—embodies this concept. We have found that this philosophy—the belief that if children *could* do well they *would* do well—helps focus staff on ascertaining *why* a child isn't doing well. Of course, in the CPS model "why" leads directly to the assessment of lagging cognitive skills.

The third major challenge is *time*, or the apparent lack of it. We say "apparent" because we find that there is often more time than school personnel think there is. But how the available time is being *used* is a different matter entirely. Nonetheless, in most schools, the schedule is not designed to provide the time necessary for the focused, ongoing discussions that are necessary to achieve a complete understanding of a student's difficulties, facilitate communication between relevant adults, permit the continuous monitoring of a child's progress, and allow for ongoing discussions about needed modifications in approach. Some school personnel aren't even aware that such in-depth discussions are necessary. There is no quick fix. There is no cookie cutter. You don't fix a reading disability in a week; you don't fix the learning disability that is explosive behavior in a week, either.

Which brings us to the final challenge: *expertise*. Most school personnel do not have a background in the cognitive factors underlying the disadvantageous behavior of children and adolescents, and have little training in and understanding of developmental psychopathology and different psychosocial and pharmacological treatment modalities. Thus, we find that school personnel tend to be eager (frequently desperate) for any information or guidance that might reduce the behavior problems of a given student, but often are wary of advice that requires changes in standard operating procedure. It is important, therefore, to "demystify" psychopathology and intervention. Once again, the CPS model requires expertise in five pathways, three plans, and the three steps for doing Plan B.

We also find that many outpatient mental health clinicians are initially uncomfortable with the idea of going to a child's school to collaborate with teachers and other staff. However, the content of discussions that take place at school *should* be quite similar to the content of discussions that take place inside the clinician's office. Of course, we italicized the word "should" in the preceding sentence because we find that in many group settings—for example, schools, inpatient units, residential facilities, or juvenile detention facilities—the information being exchanged in meetings is often of little relevance to *achieving an understanding of the cognitive underpinnings of a child's difficulties* and therefore is also of little relevance to *developing interventions that flow from this understanding*. Thus, an emphasis on situational analysis, triggers, and the pathways—discussed in prior chapters—is absolutely indispensable to helping educators understand a child's difficulties and why the child's behavior has shown little change even after countless applications of standard school discipline procedures. Our experience is that school personnel will show little enthusiasm for CPS—and are likely to "regress to the Plan A mean"—unless they fully comprehend the specific cognitive issues underlying the student's behavior problems.

Fortunately, in some respects educators are actually in the best position to understand that explosive episodes are the by-product of a learning disability, since they routinely assess, remediate, and make accommodations for other learning disabilities. On the other hand, as discussed above, because many educators have little or no background in child psychopathology and its treatments, in other respects they are not especially well equipped to understand and remediate this particular learning disability.

In initial meetings it is crucial for school personnel to share observations and information and to develop hypotheses about the factors (i.e., pathways, triggers) contributing to a student's explosive behavior. The situational analysis and Pathways Inventory should be quite helpful along these lines. It is also essential that all of the staff directly involved with the student be in attendance. It is then important to discuss the triggers or pathways that will be the initial focus of intervention, who will have initial Plan B discussions with the child, and when the next meeting will take place to discuss the child's initial response to Plan B, needed modifications to the original plan, and additional triggers or pathways that should subsequently be addressed. (By the way, in the next chapter we have included a form—called the Individualized Cognitive Challenges Plan [ICCP]—that many educators have found useful for tracking these activities.) It is likely that other explanations for the student's behavior—those related to motivation (or the lack of it), attention seeking, and manipulation—will also be raised. It's very important to question whether these instinctive explanations truly have merit:

ADULT 1: I think Johnny acts up because he doesn't want to do the work.

ADULT 2: Now, why wouldn't he want to do the work?

ADULT 1: I don't know, I guess he just doesn't feel like it.

ADULT 2: So you think he'd rather sit in the assistant principal's office?

ADULT 1: If it gets him out of doing the work, maybe.

ADULT 2: If he could do the work, don't you think he would rather stay in class and do it than get into trouble and get poor grades?

Sometimes it is strategically useful to have parents at the meeting (especially if the goal is to improve communication between parents and school personnel, gather information from parents that might be useful for clarifying lagging thinking skills, or set the stage for collaboration and continuity of care between home and school); sometimes meeting without parents makes more sense (especially if school personnel want to be comfortable speaking freely or come to a tentative set of hypotheses about pathways before involving parents in the discussion).

Achieving a consensus on lagging skills is, of course, absolutely crucial; without such a consensus, it is not possible to help those working with the student understand that (1) his explosive episodes are not manipulative, attention seeking, intentional, or due to poor motivation, but rather the by-product of a learning disability in the domains of flexibility, frustration tolerance, and problem solving; (2) that reward-and-punishment procedures are unlikely to address the cognitive deficits that are implicated in the student's difficulties; and (3) that the best chance of addressing the student's behavior problems in an effective, durable manner is to teach lacking thinking skills (just as one would with any other learning disability).

Below is an example of a dialogue from a typical first meeting (without parents present):

PRINCIPAL: Well, let's see if we can put our heads together on Sam's pathways and think about how we might be able to help him better than we are right now. (*looking at Sam's classroom teacher*) Mrs. K, why don't we start with you.

MRS. K: Where should I start?

SCHOOL PSYCHOLOGIST: I don't know him very well. And I'm no expert on the CPS model. But I think we should start with trying to figure out what his triggers and lagging skills are. What's he look like in your room? When's he having the most trouble?

MRS. K: Depends on which Sam you're talking about. He's like Jekyll and Hyde. Sometimes I look up and he's doing his work and you wouldn't even know he's in the room. Other times, he's into someone else's business and bothering people and asking to go the bathroom every 10 minutes. And if you try to set limits or talk to him about his behavior, he goes nuts. You know, he's a lot bigger than many of the other kids and when they see him getting upset I think it scares them. Scares me, too. But he doesn't seem to care about that. To tell you the truth, he doesn't seem to care how he comes across. He had a nasty episode the other day . . . laying on the ground, screaming, kicking his legs, spitting . . . I think it's the first time we've seen spitting. I was wondering if he'd had a lot of sugar that day for breakfast, or maybe just a bad morning at home.

RESOURCE ROOM TEACHER: I was there. It was like he was in a different zone!

MRS. K: You know, I'd like to help him . . . he can be a very sweet boy . . . but when he goes nuts there's no talking to him!

PRINCIPAL: Now, a few times he's become unsafe to the other children when he's been upset, and that's when I've had to get involved. I've had several phone calls from other parents about him already, and it's only November! Of course, by the time he gets to my office, he's crazed. I've learned not to even try talking to him until he's calmed down.

MRS. K: I don't like to send him down to you, but sometimes I have no choice . . . I have 26 other children in his class who I have to teach.

GUIDANCE COUNSELOR: I was reading an article about bipolar disorder last month and I was thinking to myself "That's Sam!" You know, with all the explosive episodes and everything? (*looking at school psychologist*) Do you think he has bipolar disorder?

SCHOOL PSYCHOLOGIST: I'm not quite sure what diagnosis he'd get . . . probably a bunch of 'em. But it's probably safe to say he's quite challenging to have in the classroom.

MRS. K: Oh, it's not just the classroom. It's at recess, at lunch, while waiting for the bus, during circle time . . .

PRINCIPAL: You know, his mother was telling me he fell off his bike once when he was 4 years old . . . wasn't wearing a bike helmet, of course . . . hit his head, had to go the hospital. She told us the hospital said he was fine, but I was wondering if maybe he had some sort of brain injury.

SCHOOL PSYCHOLOGIST: I'm no expert . . . but I'm not aware of any reason to think that a brain injury is coming into play, though I suppose anything's possible. I wonder what it is about recess, lunch, circle time, that are hard for Sam?

The school psychologist is trying to weed through the abundant information that has already been shared so as to keep the group focused on the important items: triggers and pathways.

RESOURCE ROOM TEACHER: I think he just doesn't want to do what he doesn't want to do. You know, it's *his* way or *no* way.

MRS. K: It's not that he's a problem every day. Some days he surprises me and does very well. Other times he's just impossible to deal with. That's what I was talking about when I said "Jekyll and Hyde."

PRINCIPAL: Mrs. K, maybe you can describe a recent explosive episode for us.

MRS. K: We had one this morning already! When we sat down for circle time, he just wouldn't settle down. He was bouncing around the room, trying to get some of the other kids going, too. We told him that he needed to join the group or else he would have to leave the class-room . . . you know, otherwise, he would disrupt circle time for the rest of the class. Then he started saying how mean I was and screaming at me! The same thing happened yesterday right after lunchtime when he refused to go to the reading corner.

SCHOOL PSYCHOLOGIST: Does that happen a lot . . . you know, does he have difficulty switching from one activity to another?

MRS. K: Yes, he's terrible with transitions. Right after recess we have the same problem. But you know, its not just transitions. He doesn't seem to grasp basic routines that have been consistent all year—like the

morning routine, even though its been the same since the first day—
you know, hang up your coat and backpack, go to your desk, take out
your journal, and open the book to today's date. Every morning I have
to remind him to put his name at the top of the new page.

SCHOOL PSYCHOLOGIST: (*looking at the Pathways Inventory*) So it sounds
like shifting from one activity to another is definitely difficult for
him, and that he's pretty hyperactive and impulsive, too. It also
sounds like there are some basic routines he still hasn't quite mastered. Any theories about what's making it hard for him while he's in
recess?

MRS. K: Well, he doesn't go to recess very often because of something that's
gone wrong before recess . . .

PRINCIPAL: It's kind of like you've got a problem no matter what you do with
him. If you let him go to recess, he's butting into other kids' games or
running into them or stealing their ball and laughing about it. If you
keep him in from recess, he's mad the rest of the day because you kept
him in from recess. But keeping him in from recess . . . well, even that
doesn't make any difference the next day, because he's back doing the
same things all over again! Doesn't seem to make a dent! Now, he's already been suspended two times this year. I was thinking we needed to
send a stronger message . . . but it didn't seem to have much impact.

GUIDANCE COUNSELOR: 'Course, you have to remember what he's going
home to.

MRS. K: Oh, I think the mom has good intentions.

SCHOOL PSYCHOLOGIST: From what I can gather, he's not exploding all the
time at school, just some of the time. That tells me that he's only exploding under certain conditions.

MRS. K: That's interesting. I've never thought about it that way.

SCHOOL PSYCHOLOGIST: Any other theories about why recess is so hard for
him?

RESOURCE ROOM TEACHER: I think he knows we can't watch him as closely in
recess so he can get away with more. That's why he hates it when we
keep him in.

MRS. K: Oh, I think he just doesn't know what to do with himself in recess . . . he reminds me of a chicken running around with his head cut
off! He just bounces from one thing to another . . .

SCHOOL PSYCHOLOGIST: And during circle time? Is that hard for the same reason?

MRS. K: Same chicken. He's told me he doesn't like circle time very much. Ask me, he can't sit still for that long. I feel bad that he can't sit still, but at some point he's got to learn that he's got to do what's expected.

GUIDANCE COUNSELOR: (*looking at the Pathways Inventory*) So that's the hyperactivity again.

Notice that the assembled are slowing starting to focus on information that is related to triggers and pathways (the group seems to be homing in on the executive pathway in particular), and focusing less on information that would head the discussion down a dead end (e.g., bipolar disorder, brain injury, he doesn't care, he's only motivated to do what he wants).

MRS. K: Well, it's not just hyperactivity. He doesn't work very well with other children . . . even when we try to pair him up with kids who still like him a little. Even Stevie—he's a little boy in our class—he gets along with everybody—but even he doesn't like working with Sam.

GUIDANCE COUNSELOR: Besides hyperactivity, are there things Sam is doing that might alienate the other kids?

MRS. K: I'll tell you the truth . . . I think we could live with the hyperactivity . . . it's the explosions that just throw the whole class for a loop. What pathway is that?

SCHOOL PSYCHOLOGIST: Well, explosive behavior isn't a pathway itself . . . the pathways are categories of skills frequently found lagging in kids who explode. Let's keep talking about other situations in which he explodes . . . maybe some other pathways will start to make sense. I think we've established that he blows up when you try to reduce his hyperactivity by setting limits. Are there other situations . . . besides limit setting . . . that cause frequent explosive episodes?

MRS. K: Things not going the way he thought they would. He just has very definite ideas about the way things are supposed to go, and when they don't go that way he falls apart.

RESOURCE ROOM TEACHER: You can say that again! He's in my room for reading. He's actually come a long way, but when something gets hard for him he immediately wants to read books that are 2 or 3 years beneath his level. I've set limits on that many times . . . and he's blown up about it many times . . . but he still does the same thing time after time. I even tried putting him on a sticker chart, but it didn't do any good.

SCHOOL PSYCHOLOGIST: Any other stories about him struggling when things don't go the way he thought they would?

MRS. K: Well, he's constantly asking to go to the bathroom. I figured that was anxiety.

SCHOOL PSYCHOLOGIST: Any theories about what he's anxious about?

RESOURCE ROOM TEACHER: Oh, I don't see him as anxious. Too clever for that.

GUIDANCE COUNSELOR: You know, it's interesting, I can't say that I see Sam as especially clever. He certainly isn't clever enough to keep himself from being punished a lot.

PRINCIPAL: That's true.

MRS. K: The other day he got upset because we had an assembly instead of recess. Is that what you mean by him getting upset about things not going the way he thought they would?

SCHOOL PSYCHOLOGIST: Maybe. Let's hear about that one.

MRS. K: Well, first of all, I don't think he even knows what time recess is. But last week we had an assembly so recess wasn't going to be until the afternoon. You would have thought the world had ended. He ended up going to neither.

PRINCIPAL: Yes, he ended up with me in the office.

SCHOOL PSYCHOLOGIST: You know, I'm looking at my Pathways Inventory, here . . . and based on what you're all saying . . . and once again, I don't know him very well . . . it sounds like there are some key lagging skills coming into play. First, it sounds like he's a very hyperactive, impulsive, disorganized kid and has a lot of trouble shifting gears. That's the executive skills pathway. I bet that's what gets in his way during circle time, recess, on the bus . . . places where he's expected to sit still and keep himself under control.

RESOURCE ROOM TEACHER: You don't think he can control that stuff?

SCHOOL PSYCHOLOGIST: Well, from what I understand, he's taking medicine that should be helping, though it sounds like we might want to talk with the mom about whether it's helping as much as it should be. I'm hoping she'll give us permission to have a conversation with the doctor doing the prescribing. But, to answer your question, no, I don't think he can control that stuff . . . otherwise—given all the times he's gotten into trouble—I think he would have stopped acting that way a long time ago.

RESOURCE ROOM TEACHER: So you don't think the punishment is helping?

SCHOOL PSYCHOLOGIST: Doesn't sound like it—isn't he still being punished for all the same things he's always been punished for?

RESOURCE ROOM TEACHER: I still think he's just doing it for attention.

GUIDANCE COUNSELOR: Oh, I think he'd like nothing more than to stop being so hyperactive, impulsive, disorganized, and explosive.

RESOURCE ROOM TEACHER: So are you saying that there shouldn't be any consequences? We do need to think about what message we're sending the other kids if he doesn't get a consequence for those things.

SCHOOL PSYCHOLOGIST: I guess I'm thinking that the other kids are waiting for us to fix the problem. They know we haven't fixed the problem yet because he's still hyperactive, impulsive, disorganized, and explosive.

RESOURCE ROOM TEACHER: But it's important for them to know we disapprove of his behavior.

SCHOOL PSYCHOLOGIST: I'm thinking they already know we disapprove of his behavior. But, as you've already said, the hyperactivity isn't even the biggest problem. Sam brings other problems to the table that makes life even tougher for him and for anyone working with him. First, it sounds like he's not very good at shifting gears from what he's thinking or doing to what we want him to be thinking or doing. Second, he's also a very concrete, black-and-white, all-or-none, literal thinker.

MRS. K: How so?

SCHOOL PSYCHOLOGIST: Well, from what you've said, it sounds like he gets an idea in his head and he can't let it go. The testing I did on him suggests that Sam isn't very good at grasping the big picture . . . when he's focused at all, he tends to focus on details. So between that and the difficulty shifting gears, he reacts very poorly to change.

MRS. K: Oh my goodness, you can say that again!

RESOURCE ROOM TEACHER: So when he's frustrated in reading he just has it in his head that he should choose an easier book?

SCHOOL PSYCHOLOGIST: Sounds like it to me. And what he's shown us is that that idea is going to stay in his head until we help him replace it with a plan that works for him.

RESOURCE ROOM TEACHER: But I've tried to replace it with another one! See this is what I don't understand about him! He knows what's going to happen to him if he chooses another book!

GUIDANCE COUNSELOR: Oh, he knows what's going to happen to him . . . but I'm not sure he knows what to do instead so it doesn't happen!

MRS. K: I'm trying to understand how these problems make him blow up.

SCHOOL PSYCHOLOGIST: Me, too. But it sounds like, because of his hyperactivity and poor impulse control, everyone's redirecting Sam a lot more often than ordinary kids. When he's redirected, he has to shift gears, and that's something he's not very good at. So he's being asked to do something he's not very good at many, many times every day and more often than most of his classmates. That's not only an interesting paradox, it's also very frustrating for him.

MRS. K: That would be frustrating.

SCHOOL PSYCHOLOGIST: So I'm betting he's experiencing the school day as much more frustrating than most kids. But the difficulty shifting gears and concrete, black-and-white thinking also make him a pretty poor problem solver. If you think about what's required for solving problems—organization, planning, figuring out what the problem is, being able to think of good ideas—he's pretty much a wash. I'd be willing to bet that when Sam is having difficulty during the school day, one of those difficulties is probably coming into play. Hyperactivity, poor planning, difficulty shifting gears, black-and-white thinking, poor problem solving.

RESOURCE ROOM TEACHER: Wow. This is a very different point of view.

MRS. K: Very different.

RESOURCE ROOM TEACHER: So what we've been doing hasn't been helping?

PRINCIPAL: It certainly hasn't fixed the problem.

SCHOOL PSYCHOLOGIST: Knowing these things about Sam makes it easier to know what we're trying to fix.

PRINCIPAL: So we're trying to fix hyperactivity, impulsiveness, poor planning . . . I forget the whole list!

SCHOOL PSYCHOLOGIST: I do think we could get more mileage out of medicine for the hyperactivity and impulsiveness part. So I'm hoping he requires less redirection once we can get that squared away. It's the rest—especially the difficulty shifting gears, concrete, black-and-white thinking, and poor problem solving—that are going to require a different approach and a lot of help from all of us and his classmates.

It's worth repeating that once a consensus has been achieved on the pathways, two important things happen: first, people stop focusing on motivational explanations for a child's disadvantageous behavior; second, people are able to home in on the precise cognitive skills that need to be trained.

SCHOOL PSYCHOLOGIST: These are hard skills to train. It's going to take a while.

MRS. K: You're not forgetting that I have 26 other kids to worry about, right?

SCHOOL PSYCHOLOGIST: Right. The good news is that . . . from what I know of the CPS model . . . this can be done in a way that doesn't take much time away from the other kids. Actually, we can probably do it in a way that sets the stage for them to help out.

MRS. K: (*laughing*) I'll take all the help I can get!

SCHOOL PSYCHOLOGIST: We've made an informal list of the situations in which Sam has the most difficulty . . . you know, the triggers. Circle time, recess, lunch, the bus, when he's working with other kids, when things don't go according to plan . . .

RESOURCE ROOM TEACHER: Sounds like the whole school day!

SCHOOL PSYCHOLOGIST: It probably feels that way. But, really, we're just dealing with a lot of problems that haven't been solved yet.

RESOURCE ROOM TEACHER: Problems that have yet to be solved?

SCHOOL PSYCHOLOGIST: Right. The reason Sam is still having these problems is that we haven't solved them yet. And he's not a very good problem solver, so he hasn't solved them yet, either! So far, all our solutions have involved trying to motivate Sam to do better or teach him that we're not happy with his behavior. But we've decided he's already motivated and he already knows we're not happy with his behavior. It's also worth pointing out that we haven't involved Sam in any of the solutions.

PRINCIPAL: I think I'm following you.

MRS. K: How do we do that?

At this point, the school staff seem to have achieved a reasonable consensus about the nature of Sam's difficulties (of course, sometimes achieving this consensus does require more than one meeting). So now would be the time to proceed with a discussion about how to translate this consensus into an action plan. Details on the how to describe the plans framework and Plan B have been provided in preceding chapters, so we don't feel the need to replicate these details here. Let's rejoin the discussion that might ensue after the basics of Plan B have been reviewed:

MRS. K: So when he starts getting upset about something I'm supposed to do the three steps . . . (reading her notes) empathy . . . define the problem . . . and invitation . . .

SCHOOL PSYCHOLOGIST: Actually, from what I've read, that would be the worst time to do Plan B.

MRS. K: (laughing) See, I'm bad at this already!

SCHOOL PSYCHOLOGIST: Well, none of us are great at it yet. It's just that there's a much better time to do Plan B than once he starts getting upset. See, we shouldn't be saving Plan B for emergencies . . . they call that Emergency Plan B. It's a bad time to do Plan B because it involves interrupting whatever your class is doing and dealing with Sam when he's already a little hot. Luckily, Sam's difficulties are highly predictable . . . we sort of know when they're coming a lot of the time . . . so we can do Proactive Plan B, which is when you or I or one of us discuss these things with him way before the problem comes up again. Same three steps . . . just better timing.

MRS. K: Well, we should have plenty of opportunity for those discussions, since he stays in from recess so often!

GUIDANCE COUNSELOR: To tell you the truth, I'm kind of hoping he's not going to be deprived of recess anymore, since we've already decided that's not working very well.

MRS. K: Oh . . . right . . . but if we're not taking away recess, what are we doing when he acts up?

GUIDANCE COUNSELOR: I think we're trying to fix the problem that caused him to act up in the first place. With Plan B.

PRINCIPAL: So if we fix the problem we won't have to keep Sam in from recess because he won't be acting up anymore.

MRS. K: Yes . . . I think I get it. So I'm supposed to find some time to have this Plan B discussion with Sam before the problem happens again . . . yes?

SCHOOL PSYCHOLOGIST: Well, I don't want you to feel like you're on your own here. We can all help out. At some point we may even be able to have some of his classmates help out. We can't tackle every problem all at once. We should take them one or two at a time. Are there some that are more important than others?

MRS. K: I'd like to tackle circle time. That is just an impossible situation . . . it gets the whole day off to a bad start. I'm in a circle with 26 other kids and Sam's causing trouble.

SCHOOL PSYCHOLOGIST: OK. So let's see if we can plow our way through the three steps. I guess empathy—using Proactive Plan B—would sound something like this: "Sam, I know it's hard for you to sit still during circle time." He's already told us that, so it's easy to empathize. Then, if we were trying to define the problem, maybe something like, "But if you wander around the room during circle time or bother the other kids, then it makes circle time very hard for the rest of us." Is that a fair summary of your concern?

MRS. K: I'd say you've captured it.

SCHOOL PSYCHOLOGIST: Next comes the invitation: "Let's think about what we can do about that" or "Can we think together about how we can solve that problem?"

MRS. K: (*writing furiously*) OK. I can try this. But what's the solution?

GUIDANCE COUNSELOR: We don't know yet . . . depends on what you guys come up with!

MRS. K: Well, to be perfectly honest, I don't care if he actually sits in the circle. I don't think he can do it. I'd be fine if he sat at a desk outside the circle. He actually seems to be interested sometimes in what the other kids are saying. I just can't have him wandering around or bothering people.

GUIDANCE COUNSELOR: Make sure he knows that. Just remember that a good solution . . . one that will stand the test of time . . . is one that addresses both concerns . . . his and yours, and is also realistic, meaning he and you can actually do what you agreed to.

MRS. K: So I can't just tell him that sitting at a desk is the solution? He has to come up with the solution?

SCHOOL PSYCHOLOGIST: I don't think it matters who comes up with the solution. And that might be the solution you settle on. But we don't know if that's the solution until we get input from Sam. There might be reasons he doesn't think your solution will work. He might have a different solution that would work better for both of you. We won't know until the conversation takes place.

MRS. K: I know Sam. He's not going to come up with anything. I mean, didn't we just all agree that part of his trouble is that he has a difficult time with problem solving in the first place?

SCHOOL PSYCHOLOGIST: Right. That's OK. So then you'll jump in and help teach him how to come up with some ideas for solutions.

MRS. K: OK, but how? I mean, I don't want to get into Plan A, right?

SCHOOL PSYCHOLOGIST: Right. But you can just throw out some tentative solutions and check them out with him.

MRS. K: What if we come up with a solution and he won't stick to his end of things?

SCHOOL PSYCHOLOGIST: I think you go back to Plan B. That's just a sign that the original solution didn't solve the problem . . . probably because it was either unrealistic or not mutually satisfactory. The good part is that if Sam is a party to the original solution he's probably going to be more invested in a discussion about why it didn't work out so well.

PRINCIPAL: Now, we should schedule another meeting a few weeks from now so we could see how things are going. There certainly are a lot of problems to solve, and we're just learning how to do this. I like the idea of knocking off each problem one at a time.

Second Meeting (2 Weeks Later)

SCHOOL PSYCHOLOGIST: So I've been hearing in dribs and drabs about how Sam is doing, but maybe you could give us all a brief summary of how things are going.

MRS. K: Well, as I told you the other day, we've had our successes and our difficult moments.

PRINCIPAL: I suspect there are many difficult moments to come. Should we start with the successes?

MRS. K: Sure. I had a very good conversation with Sam about circle time . . . which is what we said we wanted to work on after the first meeting . . . and I'm pleased to report that he's actually done quite well at sitting at a desk during circle time. He knows I'm OK with him coloring or writing while the rest of us talk, and he's even beginning to participate.

SCHOOL PSYCHOLOGIST: Wow! Sounds good! How did he respond to Plan B the first time?

MRS. K: I think he was a little shocked. I even told him we weren't going to hold him in from recess anymore . . . we need to talk about recess, by the way, because that's not going very well . . . but I think he liked Plan B. I think I'm one who was petrified!

GUIDANCE COUNSELOR: Did he have any ideas of his own for how to solve the circle-time problem?

MRS. K: No . . . the desk was the only idea either of us could come up with.

SCHOOL PSYCHOLOGIST: And it's working so far . . .

MRS. K: So far.

SCHOOL PSYCHOLOGIST: I should report that I spoke with his mom about his medication, and she agreed to talk to the doctor about it, though she didn't want us talking to the doctor directly. I think she still doesn't trust us completely. Apparently, in one of Sam's prior schools, they reported her to the state because he was missing so many days of school. Anyways, she told me that the dosage of Sam's medication has been increased, so I'm interested in hearing whether you're seeing any reduction in hyperactivity or poor impulse control in general.

MRS. K: I think it's definitely helped in the classroom but it hasn't helped in some other places. So I think we want to try to do some Plan B on some other problems.

PRINCIPAL: What's next on the agenda?

MRS. K: We've still got major problems in recess and lunch.

SCHOOL PSYCHOLOGIST: Is one causing more problems than the other?

MRS. K: Well, recess has gotten worse because until 2 weeks ago he was seldom allowed to go. He just doesn't seem to know how to play with other kids in a way that doesn't involve intruding on their games, stealing their ball. . . . I hate to say this, but it all looks pretty intentional. And I don't see how it's related to black-and-white thinking.

GUIDANCE COUNSELOR: How does it look intentional?

MRS. K: Well, he's clearly doing those things for attention.

GUIDANCE COUNSELOR: Well, if you mean that he wants the other kids to pay attention to him, then I understand what you mean. But I think he's doing those things for attention because he doesn't know how to go about getting the attention of his classmates in appropriate ways. From what I've read, a lot of concrete, black-and-white thinkers don't know how to enter a group, have trouble adjusting their approach depending on whose group they're trying to enter, and don't read social cues very well.

MRS. K: Oh, I think he'd have to be pretty clueless not to read these cues!

PRINCIPAL: You mean the other kids are being pretty clear about the fact that they want to have nothing to do with him?

MRS. K: Exactly.

SCHOOL PSYCHOLOGIST: Sounds like there are some other people we need to be doing Plan B with besides Sam.

MRS. K: Who do you mean?

SCHOOL PSYCHOLOGIST: Possibly the other kids.

MRS. K: I think they're tired of putting up with Sam. They know we'll punish them if they tease him, but that doesn't mean they want him hanging around.

SCHOOL PSYCHOLOGIST: Yes, so there's more work to be done on the classroom social scene. In fact, it's going to be hard to help Sam interact more adaptively if he's still going to be rejected by his classmates. Is that pretty much the scene in lunch as well?

MRS. K: Pretty much. No one wants to sit with him. It's not unusual for him to do something outrageous—throwing food, showing everyone the chewed-up food in his mouth, clowning around—just to get someone to look at him.

SCHOOL PSYCHOLOGIST: Well, the partial answer to those two problems—lunch and recess—is to help Sam develop more adaptive social skills. I'm wondering how Plan B can help us.

RESOURCE ROOM TEACHER: Right now, his IEP [Individualized Education Plan] is just for reading. I wonder if he needs something like a social skills group.

GUIDANCE COUNSELOR: You know, I used to do social skills groups. I guess I could get one going again. It's just that I've always found that social interactions are a two-way street. So if we don't involve his classmates—if the only one learning new skills is Sam—I'm not optimistic that things will get better.

MRS. K: Who else needs to learn skills?

GUIDANCE COUNSELOR: The other kids in his class. Sounds like they're going to need some help being open to including him again. They may also need help giving him feedback in a way he can hear. I've been reading a lot about this lately. We can talk more about it if you want.

MRS. K: How come I feel more work coming on?

GUIDANCE COUNSELOR: Well, more work now . . . less work over the long haul. But, just to make sure we're on the same page, we're talking about a two-pronged approach: social skills for Sam and social skills for the whole class.

MRS. K: I don't see how we have the time to do anything more for the entire class.

GUIDANCE COUNSELOR: Well, I'm thinking that if we can get you out of the business of putting out social brushfires, we'll actually be saving time. And there are some important social lessons for Sam's classmates to learn, too—like including others and helping out a classmate who's struggling with something.

MRS. K: I'll believe it when I see it.

PRINCIPAL: We should probably let you two discuss the classwide stuff at another time. Should we be thinking about how we can do Plan B with Sam on the lunch or recess issue?

MRS. K: Sure.

SCHOOL PSYCHOLOGIST: Take your pick.

MRS. K: Recess.

SCHOOL PSYCHOLOGIST: Well, empathy would probably sound something like—don't forget, this is Proactive B—"Sam, I've noticed that recess is really hard for you. What's up?" If we're right about Sam, he'll probably say something like "The other kids won't let me play with them." So then we'd want to empathize again: "Recess is really hard for you because the other kids won't let you play with them." Defining the problem would be something like this: "But I've noticed that some of the things you try to do to get them to play with you end up bothering them. Have you ever noticed that?" I'm very interested to hear what he says to that. Let's say he agrees. The invitation would be something like "Let's think about how we might be able to solve that problem." Maybe Sam will agree that he needs some hints from you about how to get the other kids to play with him. Maybe there's some other solution that you'll both come up with.

GUIDANCE COUNSELOR: Just remember, this is a tough skill to train, so we're going to be at this for a while. And it's going to require that we enlist his classmates. But at least with Plan B he's going to view you as his ally in dealing with this problem rather than as his enemy.

Mrs. K: I certainly don't want to be viewed as his enemy. Sometimes it's just hard to know what to do.

School psychologist: Do you feel comfortable having the conversation with him?

Mrs. K: I'll give it a whirl. I don't think I'll be as scared this time as I was on the first try!

Principal: When are we meeting again?

Note that the group continues to view Sam's difficulties as highly situational and therefore highly predictable; continues to search for common (cognitive) threads running through situations in which his difficulties arise; understands that his problems should ideally be addressed proactively, one at a time, and monitored on an ongoing basis (to assess whether agreed-upon solutions are durably solving problems); is open to the possibility that additional lagging skills or triggers have yet to be identified; and is eager to involve Sam as an active participant in the problem-solving process. Future meetings should focus on similar themes.

The school personnel with whom we work are as diverse and unique in their views and ability to understand and apply the CPS model as the families with whom we work. Regression to old mind-sets and strategies is not uncommon. However, as noted above, we are always mindful of the fact that most classroom teachers have received little if any training in childhood psychopathology and treatment. Those who have received training have often received exposure only to the operant "wing" of the social learning theory "party." Learning about and sticking to new ways of thinking and intervening requires time, patience, and perseverance. Of course, we are also mindful of the fact that "adults do well if they can, too." Thus, when we are faced with adults who have abandoned (or failed to board) the CPS ship, we are neither surprised nor alarmed. We continue to ask the same questions: "What cognitive factors are underlying the student's difficulties?"; "Is the student responding well to standard school discipline?"; "How can we solve that problem with Plan B?"

Also notice that in the above dialogue the idea that Plan B can be applied to and between classmates (and adults) has been introduced. This is another area in which many educators have limited experience and training. Let's spend some more time on this theme here.

COLLABORATIVE PROBLEM SOLVING IN GROUPS

There are a lot of good reasons to apply CPS to all the students in a classroom and school. First, learning how to resolve problems in a mutually satisfactory manner benefits *all* children and adolescents, not just those with behavior problems. Second, this learning process can set the stage for students to help one another in ways that would not be as likely without such training (and helps teachers tap into their greatest source of help in the classroom: the students themselves). Third, in every classroom, *all* students have problems that require assistance—some with flexibility and frustration tolerance, others in reading, writing, mathematics, spelling, language processing, speaking in front of a group, or making friends. This being the case, applying Plan B to the students whose difficulties are in the domains of flexibility and frustration tolerance means that such students aren't viewed or treated (in the big picture) any differently than anyone else. While full consideration of this theme is beyond the scope of this book, brief coverage is provided below.

What we mean to suggest is that the manner in which a teacher runs a classroom (and a principal runs a school) can reduce the likelihood of explosive episodes in the first place and make such outbursts easier to handle in the second place. Along these lines, we strongly advocate creating a classroom (and school) environment that (1) is accepting of individual differences and diversity, (2) emphasizes assessment of the strengths and limitations of each individual student, (3) is oriented toward community building, and (4) is committed to a "problem-solving mind-set" for students and teachers alike. What a pity that, in an era of statewide mandated testing, the emphasis is on trying to make every child look the same. Not only is this an impossible task, it also forces teachers to focus their efforts on precisely the wrong thing! The natural diversity that exists in any given classroom is the *strength* of the classroom, but only if classroom teachers (and those who help them) formulate action plans for capitalizing on one student's strengths to address another child's limitations across the totality of the school day. Children can be helped to understand (1) that "fair does not mean equal," (2) that making sure they each get what they *need* is far more important than making sure that everyone gets the exact same thing, and (3) that they will often be called upon to help each other.

A core ingredient of many such models is a daily community meeting, usually occurring at the beginning of the school day. These meetings, which typically last 30–40 minutes, provide an outstanding daily opportunity to help students learn about each other and solve problems collaboratively. Formats for and emphases of such meetings vary (see Charney, 2002; Kohn, 1996); we are particularly keen on formats that permit students to share important events in their lives and difficulties they may be having inside and outside of the classroom (followed by discussions of how classmates can be of assistance), foster discussions about the classroom community as a whole, and include subsequent discussions about how classroomwide problems can be resolved to the mutual satisfaction of the members of the community. Such meetings provide classmates with an opportunity to learn about each other and brainstorm ideas about how to be helpful. Eventually students come to the recognition that, as individuals, they have diverse strengths and limitations and that, as a group, all members are counted upon to help each other and are an important part of creating a community that is supportive of all its members. Teachers devote equal energy to creating community and to individualizing.

When difficulties do occur between students, the teacher's role is that of Plan B facilitator. Let's listen in on a typical dialogue:

SARAH: (*in a conversation with her classroom teacher, Mr. E*) I don't want to sit next to David any more during circle time.

MR. E: (*who had Sarah sitting next to David on purpose*) You don't? How come?

SARAH: I just don't want to.

MR. E: Sounds like there's a problem I should hear about. What's up?

SARAH: He annoys me.

MR. E: How so?

SARAH: He moves around so much and he's always bumping into me and I just don't want to sit next to him anymore.

MR. E: Yes, he does move around a lot, doesn't he? I didn't realize he was bothering you so much.

SARAH: Well, now you know.

MR. E: Have you tried talking to him about it?

SARAH: Yes! I've told him to stop bugging me. But he just keeps doing it.

MR. E: I wonder if he knows what you meant when you said he was bugging you. Is this something you'd like my help with?

SARAH: Yes, I want you to let me sit next to someone else.

MR. E: Well, that would be one way to handle things. But I'd like to give David the chance to try harder not to bug you.

SARAH: I already gave him the chance!

MR. E: I know you did . . . and I appreciate that you tried talking to him about it already . . . but I don't think we should give up on David yet . . . especially if there are things we could do to help him.

SARAH: Like what?

MR. E: I'm not sure yet. I think we need to talk to David about it. Do you want me to talk to him myself or do you want to be part of the discussion?

SARAH: I want you to talk to him. But I don't want him to think I was trying to get him into trouble.

MR. E: I think he knows enough about how our classroom works to know that you aren't trying to get him into trouble. But I was thinking that you might have some good ideas for how we could help David. So I was thinking it would be helpful if you were there while I'm discussing this with him, even if I do all the talking.

SARAH: Fine.

MR. E: Should we try to find a time for you and me and David to talk things over?

SARAH: OK.

Here's a transcript of the next discussion, with David, Sarah, and Mr. E:

MR. E: David, as you know, in our classroom when something is bothering somebody we try to make sure that they talk about it. As I mentioned to you yesterday, I thought it might be a good idea for me and you and Sarah to talk together about circle time.

DAVID: OK.

MR. E: Sarah's not trying to get you into trouble . . . and you're not in trouble anyway . . . but she was hoping that we could find a way for you not to have such a hard time sitting still during circle time.

DAVID: I could try harder to sit still.

MR. E: That would be very nice of you to try harder. I just wonder how long that would work, since you really do seem to have a lot of trouble sitting still during circle time.

DAVID: Yeah.

MR. E: Is there something about circle time that makes it especially hard to sit still? I noticed that you don't have quite as much trouble when you're sitting at a desk.

DAVID: It's just hard for me to sit on the ground like that . . . I don't know why . . . and when I'm at my desk I can scribble on a piece of paper so I can listen better. Plus, you let me stand up at my desk when I can't sit for very long.

MR. E: So sitting on the ground is harder for you than sitting at a desk . . . and when you're sitting at a desk you can either stand up or scribble if it's for too long.

DAVID: Yeah.

MR. E: So let's see if you and Sarah and I have any ideas about how we could make it easier for you in circle time. Do either of you have any ideas?

SARAH: Could he sit at a desk during circle time?

DAVID: Yeah! Can I?

MR. E: I don't see why not. You mean pull a desk right up to the circle so David could still be part of the group?

SARAH: That's my idea.

MR. E: It's a great idea, Sarah. Looks like you like the idea, too, David. Do you think that idea would work for you?

DAVID: We could try it.

MR. E: Well, I think it's very important to have you be a part of circle time because you're a very important member of our class . . . and if that would make it easier for you, I think we could give it a try. Now, I did want to talk about something else . . .

DAVID: Where will I sit in the circle?

MR. E: I was thinking you could sit right where you do now. But that brings up the other thing I wanted to talk about. Sometimes, when you move around a lot, you bump into people, and I was hoping you could be more careful about that.

DAVID: I could try.

MR. E: What do you think we should do if you do end up bumping into someone?

DAVID: They could remind me.

MR. E: Sarah, since you're the one who sits next to David, what do you think of the idea of reminding him if he bumps into you?

SARAH: I could, but I don't know if that will work.

MR. E: I don't know if that will work, either. If it doesn't work . . . if David keeps bumping into you, even after you've reminded him . . . let me know and we'll get back together and find a different solution. Does that work for you, Sarah?

SARAH: Yes.

MR. E: This work for you, David?

DAVID: Yup.

MR. E: OK, let's give it a try. I appreciate you guys working together to try to come up with solutions like this. Let's see how it goes.

There are a few important themes to underscore from the above dialogue. First, in a Plan B discussion between classmates, no one is "right" or "wrong," no one is blamed or "in trouble." There's no need to "send a message" or "teach a lesson." There's just a problem that needs to be solved. Second, three heads are better than one. When the seeds are sown properly, discussions among classmates about how to solve problems and consideration of how one individual can be helped by others become routine. All classmates have problems that need to be solved. All have the opportunity to help and to be helped. And all have frequent opportunities to learn how to solve problems in a mutually satisfactory manner. The teacher and other adults in the school perform the role of facilitators, not geniuses.

SCHOOLWIDE COLLABORATIVE PROBLEM SOLVING

At a schoolwide level, the CPS model has important implications for the discipline code, which tends to be a list of rules and a corresponding, rigid list of the consequences for anyone who violates the rules. While, at first glance, such lists and discipline systems might appear to have efficiency in their favor, they deserve a second look: continuing to apply consequences to students whose difficulties are not durably affected by consequences is the epitome of inefficiency, wasted effort, and futility.

Would chaos result if the discipline code were eliminated? Would the majority of the students in a school—who never have any experience with the discipline code (because the discipline code isn't why they're behaving appropriately in the first place)—begin misbehaving if the discipline code were replaced with a set of *expectations* and a "Plan B road map" for what should take place if a student is having difficulty meeting those expectations? (We favor *expectations* over *rules*, by the way, because while *rule violations* set the stage for only *one* option [Plan A], we have been quite explicit in this book about the *three* options that are available for handling *unmet expectations*: Plan A, Plan B, and Plan C.) Many school personnel often talk about the importance of "holding students accountable for their actions." It is crucial, of course, for such personnel to understand that students are being "held accountable" when one is applying Plan B.

What is a Plan B road map? It is a series of steps for helping a "problem-solving team" to (1) begin a detailed, comprehensive assessment of a student's difficulties, with an emphasis on situational factors and lagging cognitive skills contributing to these difficulties; (2) call upon outside expertise (e.g., a pediatric neuropsychologist) to further assess these difficulties, if necessary; (3) once a student's lagging cognitive skills are identified, develop an action plan, including details about which situations are to be addressed first, and which adults will be primarily responsible for implementation, including whatever Plan B discussions need to be held; and (4) decide when the problem-solving team will be meeting again to discuss the student's progress in response to the initial action plan, discuss new assessment information, and formulate adjustments to action plans in response to this new information.

Naturally, this would require some changes in standard operating procedure. As we mentioned at the beginning of this chapter, *teachers need time to talk to each other on a regular, ongoing basis.* While many schools systems appear to have recognized this need (note the increasing popularity of early release days and similar schedule changes), others continue to operate in a way that shows an utter lack of awareness of the planning and discussion that is required to formulate action plans for the many students with special needs now finding their way into general education classrooms. As we also mentioned above, teachers need *expertise* in childhood psychopathology, an understanding of the cognitive underpinnings of behavioral challenges, and an awareness of interventions flowing from this understanding. Such expertise needs to be built into the curriculum of our teacher-training programs and into programs for those already employed as teachers. Inclusion was and remains a wonderful idea, but only if we provide teachers with the tools to make the idea a good one.

Incidentally, there are many ways to build community on a *schoolwide* basis, including frequent all-school meetings (community building is a better reason to bring everyone in the school together than the fact that the football team has a game tonight). Once again, formats for such meetings vary, but all have as their foundation the desire to celebrate the community (not just the football team and cheerleaders!) and learn more about the special talents and needs of all its members (not just the quarterback or the cheerleaders!).

Finally, Plan B isn't reserved for adult–child interactions. CPS has application to adult–adult interactions as well. Indeed, whether the problems to be solved affect the entire school or those a particular teacher may be having in his or her classroom, solutions are facilitated when faculty feel comfortable talking about these difficulties among themselves, considering alternative solutions together, and therefore supporting each other. Principals demonstrate more leadership by facilitating a Plan B process in faculty meetings than by knowing all the answers.

Of course, Plan B applies to interactions between school staff and parents as well. How often we have heard parents complain of feeling misunderstood by, and uncomfortable interacting with, school personnel. How often we have heard school personnel complain that a student's parents were uncooperative and unwilling to help. It's worth noting that the definition of the word *cooperate* is "to come together, to collaborate." It's also worth remembering that the first step of Plan B is *empathy*.

We'll close this chapter with a dialogue that might take place between school personnel and the mother of Sam (the boy whose difficulties were the focus of dialogues at the beginning of this chapter):

PRINCIPAL: Thanks very much for coming in today. We were all looking forward to talking to you about Sam and how he's been doing and about how we can work together to help him even more.

SAM'S MOM: My boss wasn't too happy, but here I am.

PRINCIPAL: You know everybody around the table, yes?

SAM'S MOM: Yes, unfortunately. I don't mean I'm sorry to know you all, I mean, you know, he's always gotten into so much trouble . . .

PRINCIPAL: We understand. But I'm also pleased to report that he's getting into less trouble over the past month or so.

SAM'S MOM: Well, then you must be miracle workers!

PRINCIPAL: I don't think we're working any miracles . . . but we are trying to understand him better and involve him in helping us solve problems he encounters here.

SAM'S MOM: Any of you interested in moving into my house for a few months?

PRINCIPAL: (*laughing*) So he has his share of troubles at home, too?

SAM'S MOM: Oh, yeah. You know, his medicine wears off by the time he gets home . . . so you all have the easy Sam . . . I've got the one who can't sit still at the dinner table, goes nuts if you try to get him to quit off the computer, can't fall asleep at night, can't wake up in the morning . . .

SCHOOL PSYCHOLOGIST: Wow . . . sounds tough. Is anybody helping you with the problems you're having with Sam at home?

SAM'S MOM: Many have tried. They all tell me to do the same thing. I've probably done three dozen sticker charts with Sam.

SCHOOL PSYCHOLOGIST: The sticker charts haven't helped?

SAM'S MOM: They always work for a few weeks. Then . . . same old Sam.

SCHOOL PSYCHOLOGIST: He told me he was seeing a counselor now. Is that accurate?

SAM'S MOM: Yes, I've got him seeing a counselor at the mental health clinic. Sam likes her, but from what I can tell, all they do is play games together.

SCHOOL PSYCHOLOGIST: So you're not seeing that the counselor is helping all that much?

SAM'S MOM: Well, Sam doesn't mind going to see her like he has with some of the other counselors . . . but it's still the same old Sam.

PRINCIPAL: That must be very frustrating for you . . . to get all that help and have nothing to show for it.

SAM'S MOM: My mom—Sam's grandma—says it's like a broken arm that won't heal and doctors can't fix. So that's one of the reasons I don't like coming to these school meetings . . . all I get is bad news that I can't do anything about anyways.

GUIDANCE COUNSELOR: Does his grandma live with you?

SAM'S MOM: No, she has her own place, but she takes care of him a lot while I'm at work.

GUIDANCE COUNSELOR: We'd love to meet grandma one of these days, too.

SAM'S MOM: Oh, she's a pistol. But she's getting too old to chase after Sam.

PRINCIPAL: The good news is that we don't have a lot of bad news to report. In fact, like I said, between the changes in his medication dose and some of the things we're doing here, Sam has had a very good month.

SAM'S MOM: You know, I noticed that he's been feeling better about coming to school lately. He says you don't hold him in from recess anymore. But how come you wanted to meet with me?

SCHOOL PSYCHOLOGIST: Well, we wanted to share with you some of the things we're doing here that seem to be working better with Sam . . . so we can make sure that you're aware of what we're up to . . .

SAM'S MOM: You know what, if things are better, I'm a happy camper . . . I just hope it lasts.

SCHOOL PSYCHOLOGIST: And we also wanted to meet you because we think it's important to have a close working relationship with our parents.

SAM'S MOM: Well now there's a switch. We've had to move around a lot . . . Sam's dad was military . . . we're divorced now, of course . . . but I've never felt like the folks at school have understood how hard all this is.

SCHOOL PSYCHOLOGIST: We think Sam's a great kid, but we also see that there are also some things that make him tough. That can be very hard.

SAM'S MOM: So I haven't really been looking forward to this meeting. I mean, I don't need people helping me feel like I'm a bad parent.

SCHOOL PSYCHOLOGIST: We certainly don't want to do anything to make you feel like a bad parent. Sam has really made some good progress over the last month or two . . . things are better in recess, better at lunch, better at circle time . . .

SAM'S MOM: That's the first good news I've had about him in a long time.

SCHOOL PSYCHOLOGIST: Like I said, I think the change in his medication dosage has helped. But we did want you to know how we're going about doing things here . . . we even thought you might like to observe in the classroom if you can come in another day . . . if your boss is OK with it . . . so you can watch Sam and us in action.

SAM'S MOM: If I can get more time off, I'd love to.

SCHOOL PSYCHOLOGIST: What we're doing with Sam is trying to involve him in helping us solve some of the problems he's having here.

SAM'S MOM: He's told me something about this.

SCHOOL PSYCHOLOGIST: So Sam is now sitting at a desk during circle time . . . he's still part of the group, but he sits at a desk. And he's been eating lunch with me and some of the other kids from his class at least 3 days a week. That was his idea. We feel it's given him a nice chance to connect with some of the kids in the class under controlled circumstances.

SAM'S MOM: He told me something about that, too. Here I thought that meant he was in trouble.

SCHOOL PSYCHOLOGIST: No, he's not in trouble. Quite the opposite. We've noticed that he's doing a little better in recess because of some of the connections he's made with other kids during lunch group. Of course, we've done some work with all the kids in the class to help them all get along better with each other.

PRINCIPAL: We're very happy with how much progress he's made in a very short period of time. Mrs. K, you've been very quiet. Perhaps you can tell us how Sam's been looking lately in the classroom.

MRS. K: He's better. Believe me, he still has some trouble staying still and paying attention, but he's doing better. He and I are trying hard to work on some of those problems. One of the things I've noticed is that he almost never has his homework done, and that's one of the things we thought we could talk with you about.

SAM'S MOM: I know. I'm sorry.

PRINCIPAL: Oh, no need to be sorry. We just want to understand the problem so we can think about how to approach it.

SAM'S MOM: See, I don't get home until 8:00 P.M. . . . sometimes I can catch a ride and get home earlier, but mostly I have to take the bus and it takes forever. So, like I said, my mom watches him, but I don't think she's going to be able to get him to do his homework. And by the time I get home . . . I mean, I hate to say this . . . but I'm exhausted.

SCHOOL PSYCHOLOGIST: I understand.

SAM'S MOM: Plus, he never brings home what he needs to do the homework anyway.

MRS. K: I could check his backpack at the end of every day to make sure he has what he needs.

SCHOOL PSYCHOLOGIST: That could help . . . on the other hand, it sounds like even if Sam had what he needed it would be very hard for him to complete his homework.

SAM'S MOM: I'm sorry. I could try harder. I just don't want to make any promises I can't keep.

PRINCIPAL: Really, there's nothing to be sorry about. We were just hoping we could put our heads together to try to solve the problem. Mrs. K, how important is it that Sam complete homework?

MRS. K: Well, most of what I give for homework is practice . . . so he's missing out on some practice by not doing it. I don't think that's such a big deal. Do you think we should just dispense with the homework expectation for Sam?

SCHOOL PSYCHOLOGIST: That's one option.

MRS. K: The only problem I have with that is that the homework expectations increase a lot next year. So we may not be doing him any favors by telling him he doesn't have to do his homework this year. Plus, I wonder what his classmates are going to think of his not doing any homework.

GUIDANCE COUNSELOR: Well, I'm betting that the work we're doing now with all the kids in the class—especially around the theme that fair doesn't mean equal—will take care of the latter concern . . . if he ends up doing no homework, that is.

SAM'S MOM: I don't even know how much homework he gets every night, so I don't know how much homework he's not doing.

MRS. K: Well, I usually give 30–45 minutes of homework a night. And I want you to know that Sam's not the only one who isn't doing all his homework.

PRINCIPAL: If Sam's mom thinks she might be able to get him to do maybe 10 minutes of homework a night, maybe we could prioritize the assignments. But, under the circumstances, maybe even 10 minutes isn't realistic.

SAM'S MOM: I could get him to do 10 minutes of homework a night if there's a way for me to know exactly what he's supposed to be doing and you all could make sure the right assignments get home.

SCHOOL PSYCHOLOGIST: Are you sure? Because I don't think any of us is thinking that homework is a huge deal right now. We understand how exhausted you must be.

SAM'S MOM: No, no, if I know what he's supposed to do and it's only 10 minutes and he's got the right materials, I'll get him to do it. I don't want to give up on homework completely.

MRS. K: I can check his backpack before he leaves every day . . . don't we need to check this arrangement out with Sam?

SCHOOL PSYCHOLOGIST: Good point. I can talk to him about it tomorrow. Let's assume he'll be OK with it. How are we going to make sure that Mom knows what Sam's supposed to be doing?

MRS. K: (to Sam's mom) Do you get email?

SAM'S MOM: I do. Sam taught me how to check it.

MRS. K: (*to Sam's mom*) I'll email you with his assignments every day.

PRINCIPAL: (*to Mrs. K*) You're sure you can do this every day?

MRS. K: It's not a problem. I'm actually thinking Sam might be able to help me with that.

PRINCIPAL: Fantastic!

SCHOOL PSYCHOLOGIST: Sounds like a plan. (*to Sam's mom*) Now, if you run into any trouble with this plan, please let us know. We'll figure out a new plan. I'll give you my direct line before you leave.

SAM'S MOM: Now, this plan will work most nights. But some nights I have to work overtime and I won't be able to make sure he does his homework.

SCHOOL PSYCHOLOGIST: We'll assume if the homework doesn't come in the next day that you had to work late. But let us know if you run into trouble on the nights you don't work late.

SAM'S MOM: Will he get a zero if the homework doesn't come in?

PRINCIPAL: I think that for now . . . and I've already talked with Mrs. K about this . . . homework isn't going to affect Sam's grades.

SCHOOL PSYCHOLOGIST: Before we end, there is one other thing we wanted to talk about.

SAM'S MOM: Uh-oh.

SCHOOL PSYCHOLOGIST: No, nothing bad. It's just that, in the same way that we want to work together with you to help Sam, we also like to work with other people outside the school who are also working with him. I know you've had a bad experience with this, but it would be very helpful if we could communicate directly with the doctor prescribing his medicine and with the counselor he's seeing. We just hate to trouble you every time we want to let the doctor know what we're seeing here at school.

SAM'S MOM: Um . . . I'll have to think about that one. Like what kind of things would you be talking about?

SCHOOL PSYCHOLOGIST: Well, with the counselor, we'd like to make sure that everyone's on the same page in working with Sam and get a sense for how she's viewing his difficulties. With the doctor who's prescribing the medicine, we'd just like to share our observations about how the medicine is working.

SAM'S MOM: So, like, are you all going to tell him what to do with the medicine? Is he going to change the medicine without me knowing about it?

SCHOOL PSYCHOLOGIST: We are not the medicine experts . . . your doctor is . . . we just want to make sure he's got the most current information about how Sam is doing.

SAM'S MOM: I really need to think about this. You all seem like good people . . . and you seem to understand Sam . . . but I don't know if I'm comfortable enough to have you talking directly to his doctor about the medicine. I don't have a problem with the counselor coming to a meeting here, but I'd want to be here, too.

PRINCIPAL: That's not a problem. We don't want you to be uncomfortable, and you're right, you don't know us very well yet. Maybe we should schedule another meeting and we can make it at a time that's convenient for you and the counselor. And, until you're comfortable, we'll keep communicating with the doctor through you.

SAM'S MOM: I don't want you all thinking I'm paranoid or anything . . . I don't have anything to hide . . . it's just that I'm not that comfortable with Sam being on medicine in the first place . . . we've had some bad experiences with medicine . . . so I want to make sure I know exactly what's going on.

PRINCIPAL: I understand completely. I'm very comfortable with the plan we've got. If your comfort level increases once you know us a little better, or if there's another way for us to communicate with the doctor that makes you more comfortable, just let us know. I was wondering if you had any concerns you wanted to make sure we talk about while you're here.

SAM'S MOM: No . . . none that I can think of.

PRINCIPAL: Well, then I really want to thank you for coming in today. I know it wasn't easy for you. But I think we're off to a good start.

SAM'S MOM: Thank you all so much. I'm sorry he gives you so much trouble.

SCHOOL PSYCHOLOGIST: Well, we like having him here. He's a great kid. We've just got some problems to solve and it's nice to know that we can work with you and Sam to solve them.

Q & A

What if you've done your best and you simply can't get the child's parents to work with you? How important is it that application of the CPS model be consistent between home and school?

Achieving consistency between home and school is the ideal. Sometimes, the main reason such consistency has not been achieved is because the parties didn't first achieve a consensus on the explanation for the child's difficulties and therefore disagree completely on what to do about the problem that remains ill defined. Sometimes it's not possible to achieve the ideal. Keep trying. And remember that the first step of Plan B is empathy. In the meantime, recognize that school personnel are still on the hook for doing the right thing for the 6 hours a day and 9 months of the year that the child is in their hands. The only other option, of course, is to do the wrong thing in the spirit of consistency, which makes no sense whatsoever.

In saying that explosive behavior is a learning disability, are you implying that these children always require involvement in special education?

Hardly. There are some lagging skills that might require help from special education, such as language-processing skills. Others, such as social skills, might not require special education assistance. So we don't think all of these children will need help from special education. Some might not even require a 504 plan. More than anything, what they are need is a talented teacher who (we hope) knows something about the five pathways, the three plans, and the three steps for doing Plan B.

Can Plan B be written into an IEP?

Absolutely. Indeed, to the degree that an IEP is intended to state explicitly how a child's difficulties are to be handled, we actually think it's a good idea to have Plan B "codified" in the IEP. As we mentioned earlier in the chapter, we've also developed a form—called the Individualized Cognitive Challenges Plan (ICCP)—to help track the lagging skills and triggers that are the present focus of intervention. The ICCP is included in the next chapter.

Chapter 8

Collaborative Problem Solving in Therapeutic/Restrictive Settings

Implementing CPS in restrictive therapeutic settings (e.g., inpatient units, therapeutic day schools, residential and juvenile detention facilities) can be extraordinarily challenging because *all* the youths being served have significant needs—with many exhibiting violent, destructive, aggressive behavior—and perhaps especially because many such settings have a long-standing commitment to Plan A as the primary mode of intervention. While the challenge is undeniably daunting, implementation of CPS can raise standards of care and help achieve the foremost goal of intervention: *ensuring that a child has learned the cognitive skills necessary to obviate the need for continued placement in the facility.* All of the elements presented in earlier chapters—assessing and identifying lagging cognitive skills, analysis of situational factors contributing to maladaptive behavior, the plans framework, and the steps for and difficulties associated with implementing Plan B—have application to therapeutic facilities. Because examples of Plan B dialogues and the contrasting tones and language of Plans A, B, and C have been provided in preceding chapters, we do not provide such examples in this chapter. Rather,

187

we focus on the special considerations that come into play when implementing CPS in these facilities.

It is not surprising that staff in restrictive settings tends to rely heavily on Plan A, often in the form of a level system. In many such settings, the training staff are provided tends to be oriented toward implementation of a contingency management program, which is relied upon to achieve consistency of approach across staff. We find that such consistency is, in fact, rarely achieved, with some staff working hard to establish relationships and to communicate with residents and other staff demonstrating facility only with the mathematics of the point and level system, the issuing of clear commands, and the algorithm of rewards and punishments. On some units, turnover is quite high, so achieving consistency and continuity across shifts and over weeks and months is extremely difficult. When a resident is not responding optimally to the incentive program, there is often a tendency to try to "improve the wheel," which generally translates into more "meaningful" or painful punishments. When asked about potential changes that might lead to improvements in their settings, it is common for some staff members to reply, "I think what we really need is a better motivational system. We just haven't found the best way to motivate these kids yet." We are reminded of the adage "If the only tool in your toolbox is a hammer, you will treat everything as though it is a nail."

Fortunately, receptivity to the CPS model in such settings is growing due to the admirable national initiative to reduce chemical, physical, and mechanical restraint and locked-door seclusion. Along these lines, a majority of the youth who find their way into such settings have abuse histories, and therefore restraint and seclusion (R/S) procedures would be the last thing we'd want such youth to experience (or witness) in a "safe" setting. But let us be clear from the outset: while reduction in restraint and seclusion is a worthy end in itself, it is most effectively understood and pursued as a by-product of good care.

In our intensive consultation work with numerous therapeutic facilities, we have found that there is often no existing mechanism for reconciling disparate staff conceptions of the maladaptive behavior of residents. In its emphasis on the cognitive underpinnings of maladaptive behavior, the CPS model can help staff achieve a level of insight into such behavior that they may not have previously possessed. Further, there is often an utter lack of communication and collaboration within and between clinical staff and milieu staff. Indeed, in many settings, milieu staff is relegated to the role of "baby-sitter," with the "really important work" left to the clinical staff. In its emphasis on pathways, triggers, and the plans framework, the CPS model can help *all* staff communicate

more effectively about assessment information and collaborate on intervention so that *all* staff members are in a position to do really important work with
the residents.

But perhaps most importantly, we have observed that, similar to schools,
it is rare for such settings to have a *philosophy* about children. If there is a
guiding belief system in such settings, it is that reward-and-punishment programs must be employed to provide structure and to control behavior (this
mentality can be the by-product of both the behavioral and the psychoanalytic
perspectives). We find that *"Children do well if they can"* is as important a
guiding philosophy in restrictive settings as it is in any other setting. Along
these lines, we often ask staff in such facilities to contrast the mentality they
tend to apply to an explosive child with the mentality they would apply to a
psychotic child; they are often surprised by the disparity.

SLOWLY MOVING FROM A TO B

First and foremost, initiation of CPS requires significant support from directors
and administrators, for the purposes of serving as role models for learning the
new approach and to ensure "intestinal fortitude" to see the unit through the difficult times that are to be expected during such a significant transition in unit
culture and practice. Leadership must have a clear vision about the type of environment they are trying to create and a clear definition of the word *therapeutic*.

If a facility is truly dedicated to implementation of the CPS model, a
mechanism for ongoing supervision must be put into place. Providing staff
with a one-time overview of the pathways and the plans framework is utterly
insufficient if CPS is to be implemented in a comprehensive manner. Why?
First, no one feels competent at assessing pathways and implementing Plan B
after one exposure to the material. Second, once staff become familiar with the
plans framework, life gets much more interesting. Staff members who have
been unofficially operating from a Plan B framework all along feel vindicated.
But staff members who have been relying heavily on Plan A now find that their
modus operandi is being challenged. Because some of these staff members do
not yet feel confident in their Plan B skills—or have been operating on the assumption that "Plan A" and "having expectations" are synonymous—they often feel that dropping all expectations (Plan C) is their only remaining option.
This can lead to a deterioration in the overall stability of the facility and, understandably, to considerable discomfort, frustration, anger, and, in some
cases, attrition in staff. Other staff members may stick around but quietly (or

sometimes not so quietly) attempt to undermine the changes taking place on the unit. The hope, of course, is that these staff members will be willing to express their concerns in ongoing supervision so that their concerns can be addressed and new Plan B skills can be trained. In supervision sessions, additional guidance, support, and understanding are provided to staff members who are having difficulty adapting to and integrating the new model of care. Some units have found it necessary to have additional staff meetings separate from supervision to provide such support.

During the early phases of implementing CPS, we do not typically encourage total discontinuation of the existing contingency management program. Rather, we encourage ongoing discussion of how problems or unmet expectations that were handled with Plan A could have instead been handled with Plan B (preferably proactively), and try to practice how Plan B dialogues might have sounded. Our experience is that when staff feels comfortable enough using CPS as a means of solving problems and preventing escalation, the behavior management program "rusts away," typically through lack of use, and becomes obsolete.

Of course, the fact that Plan A is the most common *precursor* to explosive episodes is also quite convincing. Indeed, we find that when we "rewind the tape" of an explosive episode back to its genesis, it is *staff demands over minor issues that are typically implicated.* In other words, explosive episodes frequently follow a very common pattern: (1) a staff member observes a resident exhibiting an inappropriate behavior ("I'm not eating this crap for breakfast!"); (2) the staff member issues a command in an effort to stop the inappropriate behavior or to remind the resident of the rules ("Number one, that's inappropriate language and, number two, that's what's for breakfast"); (3) the resident becomes more agitated ("It sucks—I'm not eating it!"); (4) the staff member reminds the resident of the consequences of noncompliance, that is, a reduction in level and corresponding loss of privileges ("If you don't stop swearing, you're going to lose your points"); (5) the resident becomes more agitated and his or her behavior worsens or intensifies (throwing the food tray on the floor and stating, "I don't give a damn what you do to me, I'm not eating that crap!"); (6) the staff member confirms the promised loss of points ("You just lost 2 points—now go to your room!") as other staff, having heard the commotion, arrive on the scene; (7) the resident, now both far more aroused and far less capable of rational thought, does something irrational (tipping over a chair or table); and (8) the staff, now both far more aroused and far less capable of rational thought, restrains the resident (or worse).

Again, one of the most important uses of ongoing supervision is to "replay" such scenarios so that staff can consider what might have ensued had

Emergency Plan B been applied instead of Plan A: (1) the staff member would have observed a resident exhibiting an inappropriate behavior ("I'm not eating this crap for breakfast!"); (2) the staff member would have attempted to empathize or seek clarification ("You're not eating the French toast for breakfast . . . what's up?"); (3) the resident would have clarified his or her concern ("I don't like French toast"); (4) the staff member would have reempathized, placed a corresponding concern on the table, and invited the resident to solve the problem collaboratively ("You don't like French toast . . . and that's what they brought for breakfast . . . let's think of what we can do about that"); (5) the problem is solved in a mutually satisfactory manner ("We could see if there's anything in the kitchen—would cereal work for you if we can scare some up?"). When their concerns are taken seriously, the threat of formal consequences is removed from the equation, and with the knowledge that staff is trying to understand, be responsive, and help solve the problem, residents are typically able to maintain coherence, avoid cognitive debilitation, and engage in a discussion aimed at solving the problem at hand. Of course, if staff feel that a problem that was handled with Emergency B is not durably resolved, it is crucial that a subsequent Proactive B discussion take place for the purpose of working toward a more durable solution.

Two important points can be made about the above scenario. First, there are some staff members who will feel that teaching a resident to comply with adult directives (or other "life lessons") is the foremost goal during the resident's stay in the facility, safe in the assumption that those responsible for the resident's care prior to admission simply botched the job. Such staff members may justify their use of Plan A as follows: "In the real world, you can't always eat what you want." While this latter point has its merits, it is probably worth pointing out that *therapeutic facilities do not and cannot replicate the real world anyway*. The real world does not have a 5:1 staffing ratio, 24-hour supervision, and constant reminders about and enforcement of the consequences of one's actions. We are reminded of the words of an adolescent who was returned to a juvenile detention facility only 2 months after being discharged. When asked what went wrong, he responded, "I didn't have you guys [the staff] telling me what to do anymore and making sure I did it." Thus, our mantra (especially for longer stay facilities) is: "If you don't teach lacking thinking skills while the resident is in your facility, keep your door open because he's coming back."

Second—and just as important—there is an outstanding likelihood that the scenario (and coinciding explosive episode) was, in fact, *highly predictable*. In other words, it is likely that there had been several prior outbursts over the exact same problem, and therefore that the scenario simply represents a "problem that has yet to be solved." Thus, it wouldn't have been necessary to use Emergency Plan B if staff had engaged the resident in Proactive Plan B prior to the scenario recurring. For this to occur, of course, it is often necessary to greatly improve mechanisms for communicating and collaborating among all staff, an issue that is addressed more fully in the following pages.

CHANGING THE ROLE OF MILIEU STAFF

The above discussion makes clear that the CPS model elevates and expands the role of milieu staff, from enforcer of rules and point arbiter to *observer* (of the resident's interactions and behaviors), *assessor* (of the cognitive factors underlying the resident's difficulties), *problem solver* (collaboratively, of course), and (length of stay permitting) *teacher* (of lacking thinking skills). Length of stay ultimately determines whether staff has the opportunity to move beyond observation and assessment and actually address and remediate the cognitive factors underlying a resident's difficulties. For example, on an inpatient unit where the average length of stay is 1–4 weeks, stabilization and observation/assessment will be the primary goals, facilitating informed guidance regarding the resident's next placement (which is where most of the actual follow-up skills training will be accomplished). Indeed, we find that one of the greatest challenges for staff in short-stay facilities is confronting the reality that they can't "fix everything" about a resident in 1–4 weeks. In fact, they can't fix *most* things in 1–4 weeks. But they *can* do an excellent assessment of pathways and triggers, gauge a child's initial response to skills training on a few pathways or Plan B on a few triggers, and write a discharge summary that is heavy on pinpointing lagging thinking skills and that de-emphasizes diagnostic classification. If a resident is "stuck" on an inpatient unit, and therefore has a significantly longer length of stay, the stage is set for more skills training to occur (likely length of stay, of course, is not always known at admission). Length of stay in residential and juvenile detention facilities and therapeutic day schools is typically measured in months rather than weeks; this means that more skills training should occur in these settings.

To be fair—perhaps this is a statement of the obvious—not all explosive episodes are predictable. On one child inpatient unit, a resident who was otherwise reasonably engaged in the milieu was told on the telephone by his caseworker that the decision had been made to place him in a residential facility rather than allow him to return home to live with his parents. This extremely disappointing news precipitated an explosive outburst that had nothing whatsoever to do with staff or the unit. As the boy acted out his anger and frustration—by screaming, tipping over tables, and banging his fists into walls—staff moved other residents into a different part of the unit to ensure their safety and valiantly tried to help the boy express his anger without jeopardizing his or staff members' safety. Of course, staff could have elected to simply restrain the boy to ensure his and their safety, but a concerted effort was made to avoid this course of action. The episode lasted for over an hour. Staff finally helped the boy calm down. In supervision several days later, staff recounted how difficult the episode had been. Like all supervision sessions, the agenda is to validate staff concerns (empathy), revisit the goals of the unit (What are we trying to accomplish?), reconsider the relative merits of different approaches (Plans A and B) to the same problem, and correct misperceptions about the CPS model:

STAFF MEMBER 1: I want to know if we did the right thing the other day with Davis.

STAFF MEMBER 2: Geez, that was intense. Luckily nobody got hurt.

STAFF MEMBER 3: I wasn't here . . . what happened?

CHARGE NURSE: Davis's caseworker—a real genius, I might add—told him he wasn't going home. Of course, she gave us no warning whatsoever that she was going to give him that news. Can you imagine?

STAFF MEMBER 3: Where's he going?

UNIT PSYCHOLOGIST:: To a residential facility.

STAFF MEMBER 3: How'd he take the news?

STAFF MEMBER 1: Badly. Very badly. He was tipping over chairs, banging his fists into walls, screaming. It went on for a long time.

STAFF MEMBER 3: What did you all do?

CHARGE NURSE: Well, some of us herded all the other kids into the other end of the unit. Luckily, everybody went. Others of us tried to calm him down.

STAFF MEMBER 2: Let me tell you, it wasn't easy watching him do that stuff without laying hands on.

STAFF MEMBER 3: How come you guys didn't lay hands on?

STAFF MEMBER 1: Because we're trying hard not to do that anymore! Plus, poor kid finds out he's not going home, the last thing I want to do is jump on him. I just want to know if we're doing the right thing by letting him go nuts like that.

STAFF PSYCHOLOGIST: Well, it's not like we all just stood around and let him go nuts. We tried to talk him down, and eventually we actually did. And nobody got hurt . . . that's a good thing.

CHARGE NURSE: I was really proud of how everybody hung in there with him. I think Davis really appreciated that once he calmed down.

MEDICAL DIRECTOR: But why are you guys wondering if you did the right thing?

UNIT NURSE: Look, I've been keeping my mouth shut, but we're supposed to talk about how we feel in here, right?

MEDICAL DIRECTOR: Right.

UNIT NURSE: That was my license on the line during that episode, and I thought he should have been restrained. A prn would have calmed him right down and we wouldn't have had to go through all this Plan B crap to make it happen. I'm sorry, but if he hurt himself or one of the staff or other kids during this episode, I'm the one who loses my license. I mean, he's on this unit so we can help him be safe, right?

STAFF MEMBER 1: That's why I want to know if we did the right thing.

STAFF PSYCHOLOGIST: Well, you know, as we continue trying to implement CPS, we may find that there are times when Plan A and restraint are still going to be necessary. I guess I'm wondering if this would have gone any differently had Davis been restrained. In other words, would the situation have been handled better if we'd done things the old way?

STAFF MEMBER 1: Well, the episode sure as hell wouldn't have lasted an hour, that's for sure.

STAFF MEMBER 2: Yeah, but what would we have accomplished that would have been any better? None of us got hurt. The other kids were safe. Davis didn't get hurt. So he went nuts for an hour . . . and for a good reason, too . . . and we were able to calm him down without jumping on him. Isn't that what we're really here for?

CHARGE NURSE: I agree. I mean, it was intense trying to calm him down without restraining him. But it would have been intense if we'd jumped on him, too. Intense is part of the program around here. Every day is intense. If intense is not your cup of tea, then this may not be your ideal workplace. But I'll tell you what—that episode would've been a heckuva lot worse if we'd laid hands on him. And what message would we have sent him? That we don't understand . . . that we can't handle his intense feelings. As intense as it was, I think it would've been a lot worse the old way.

STAFF MEMBER 1: But what message are we sending him if we let him get away with tipping chairs over, banging his fists into walls, screaming . . .

STAFF MEMBER 2: Well, I was talking to him that same night . . . this was after he'd calmed down . . . and he told me that on other units he's been on they would have laid him out flat in a minute for that stuff. He told me how glad he was that we don't do that here.

STAFF MEMBER 1: OK, so it was better for Davis, but what message are we sending the other kids when they see him getting away with that stuff?

UNIT NURSE: Good question.

CHARGE NURSE: What message are you sending them if you restrain him or lock him in a room? Most of these kids have trauma histories . . . don't forget, Davis has a bad trauma history . . . why on earth would we want to restrain him or give him a prn if we could calm him down another way?

STAFF MEMBER 1: Look, the other day the new kid, Justin, was taunting me, saying, "Ha ha, we can do anything we want around here because you guys can't restrain us." What message does that send the other kids?

MEDICAL DIRECTOR: What did you say to Justin?

STAFF MEMBER 1: I didn't know what to say.

MEDICAL DIRECTOR: Well, first of all, the fact that you're trying not to use Plan A or restraint anymore doesn't mean the kids can do anything they want. Using Plan B doesn't mean we've dropped our expectations. But you might have said something like, "That's right, we don't restrain kids around here because we don't think it's the right thing to do. And from what I can tell, you kids don't think it's the right thing to do, either. So maybe you've been on other units where they've done that sort of thing, but we think this is a much nicer, safer place for you to work on your problems because we don't do those things here."

UNIT NURSE: So there's no limit setting around here anymore? Anything goes?

STAFF PSYCHOLOGIST: I don't see where anyone has said anything goes. You're setting limits with Plan B, too. But when you set limits with Plan B, you're doing it in way that reduces the likelihood of explosive episodes and increases the likelihood that Davis is going to seek you out next time he's bummed out about something else that happens to him around here. Plan B helps you build relationships with kids that serve you well next time things get hairy. But doing Plan B doesn't give him the message that it's OK for him to go nuts.

UNIT NURSE: Look, maybe I'm missing something, but I believe in holding kids accountable for their actions. That's the way things work in the real world.

STAFF PSYCHOLOGIST: I believe in holding kids accountable, too. Plan A isn't the only way to hold a kid accountable. You're holding kids accountable with Plan B, too, but in a different way. If they're taking your concerns about their behavior into account and working with you to find mutually satisfactory solutions so the behavior doesn't occur anymore, I'd say they're being held accountable.

UNIT NURSE: This definitely takes some getting used to. That was very scary the other day.

CHARGE NURSE: Hey, I was there, too. And I was scared, too. It does take some getting used to. But I think we did an incredible job the other day.

As the above dialogue suggests, staff typically have important concerns about whether they're "giving in" by using Plan B, whether the wrong behaviors are being reinforced, and whether other residents are being given the "wrong message." Again, supervision is where these concerns are heard and discussed. Perhaps another dialogue will help, this one from an adolescent inpatient unit.

UNIT NURSE 1: I was hoping we could use today's meeting to discuss how I used Plan B the other day with Manny. I'm hearing that a lot of people were concerned that I gave him the wrong message.

STAFF PSYCHOLOGIST: Sounds like a good use of our time.

UNIT NURSE 1: Well, as some of you have heard, Manny and a few of the other boys were threatening to have a riot over the weekend. So I decided to try Plan B . . . you know, see if I could get anywhere with him and prevent a riot.

STAFF MEMBER 1: I heard about this.

UNIT NURSE 1: So anyway, I tried talking to him about it . . . you know, proactively.

MEDICAL DIRECTOR: What did you say?

UNIT NURSE 1: I said something like, "I heard you were talking about starting a riot. What's up?"

STAFF PSYCHOLOGIST: That's a good example of trying to get a kid's concern on the table instead of his solution.

STAFF MEMBER 2: I don't understand.

STAFF PSYCHOLOGIST: Well, throwing a riot is a solution to a concern, not a concern.

STAFF MEMBER 2: Gotcha.

UNIT NURSE 1: So he told me that he wanted to have a riot as a way of saying good-bye to Pedro, who was being discharged in a few days. I thought Manny and I had a very good discussion about how there might be other ways to give Pedro a nice send-off without tearing the unit apart. I suggested that we have a good-bye party and get cookies and stuff. Manny was thinking pizza, and I said OK to that. He was also thinking he only wanted four of the boys on the unit to be invited to the party, and I told him that I thought that might make a lot of the other kids feel bad, so he agreed that everyone could be invited. So we had the pizza party and there was no riot.

MEDICAL DIRECTOR: So what are people upset about?

STAFF MEMBER 2: I think a lot of people are feeling like Manny got rewarded for threatening to riot . . . that he was just being manipulative.

UNIT NURSE 2: I'm one of those people. I mean, what are we going to do, throw a pizza party every time one of the kids threatens to riot?

STAFF PSYCHOLOGIST: I guess it would make sense to me that Manny was being manipulative if what he wanted was a pizza party. But the party wasn't even his idea. His idea was that the best way to give Pedro an appropriate send-off was to have a riot. What he learned is that staff will help him figure out what his concern is and that they'll listen to him. He learned that we'll help him come up with something more adaptive than his original plan. We found out that Manny is actually receptive to this sort of thing. And there was no riot . . . no one got hurt, no property got destroyed, no one got restrained. His concern was addressed . . . our concern was addressed. Sounds like a very positive outcome all the way around.

STAFF MEMBER 1: Oh, I didn't know the whole story. I didn't know that's why he wanted to have a riot.

UNIT NURSE 2: What if we couldn't do pizza? What if that wasn't feasible?

CHARGE NURSE: Then there would have been more to talk about with Plan B.

MEDICAL DIRECTOR: Truth is, we can't afford to have a pizza party on this unit every time someone gets discharged. But if the kids want to have a send-off for someone, we're always willing to talk about it.

STAFF PSYCHOLOGIST: And the next time Manny says he wants to riot, because we did Plan B this time, we can say to him, "Manny, last time you said you wanted to riot it was because you wanted to give Pedro a nice send-off. Maybe you could tell us what's concerning you, but this time without the rioting part."

PATHWAYS, PATHWAYS, PATHWAYS

As discussed in previous chapters, explosive episodes can also be viewed as assessment opportunities. Was any new information provided by the outburst? What factors set the outburst in motion? A specific trigger? A lacking cognitive skill? A staff member using Plan A? Ultimately, our goal is to move on to other important questions: How are we going to prevent the next explosive episode? Do we need to adjust our expectations for this resident? Has the problem that precipitated the outbursts been solved? Are there additional lacking thinking skills to be trained? How can we increase the likelihood that Plan B will be utilized by the staff member the next time?

In supervision sessions, staff members are typically asked to identify a resident whose difficulties are of particular concern or negatively impacting the overall milieu. As described in earlier chapters, the emphasis is on identifying the triggers that are precipitating explosive episodes and on identifying the lagging cognitive skills that are setting the stage for such episodes. This emphasis has a dual purpose: (1) to achieve a significantly clearer understanding of one resident's difficulties; and (2) to learn how to apply the same thinking process and understanding to *other* residents so that Plan B isn't implemented "blindly." In other words, as we've discussed elsewhere, while there are clear advantages to having staff deal with unmet expectations with Plan B instead of Plan A, the CPS model is even more effective when each child's lagging skills have been identified and staff are aware of the specific cognitive skills they are trying to train in each resident. Otherwise there is the risk that staff is doing a lot of Plan B and preventing many explosive episodes but the residents are acquiring no new thinking skills.

As when working with parents and teachers, it is absolutely crucial to help staff remain focused on the pathways. We find that in most staff meetings there is an abundance of "theories" that might explain a resident's behavior and many, many details that could be discussed, most of which have no relevance whatsoever to the pathways, to problems yet to be solved, or to how we're hoping milieu staff members will begin to interact with the resident. In other words, it is crucial that information gathered and shared in supervision be translatable and translated into an action plan—otherwise, milieu staff never escape the role of baby-sitter. And we recommend a short timeline (perhaps 3 days) on beginning the process of hypothesizing about a resident's pathways.

CHARGE NURSE: Can we talk about Tyrone today? I feel like everybody's walking on eggshells around him.

STAFF MEMBER 1: Is that the new admission? I haven't met him yet.

STAFF NURSE: Yes, he was admitted Saturday night . . . I did the admission. He tried to strangle his grandmother . . . that's who he lives with.

SOCIAL WORKER: I've got some other information about him. I talked to the guidance counselor at his current school. His biological mother was a prostitute and was using crack while she was pregnant with Tyrone. No one knows who his father was. He was in and out of foster care . . . eventually his grandmother got him. He has a history of physical abuse and maybe sexual abuse. By the fourth grade, the grandmother was having trouble getting him to go to school; when he did go he was hyperactive, lots of fights with other kids, lots of explosions. From what I hear, they've passed him every year because they don't think keeping him back will do him any good. So the school system placed him in a therapeutic day school for the fifth grade last year. His grandmother still can't get him to go. Ask me, the school system is just sitting on it because they know the grandmother doesn't know how to advocate for him. Of course, he's awfully young for a residential placement . . .

MEDICAL DIRECTOR: That's very interesting background information. Let's see if we can get a handle on what lagging thinking skills may be coming into play. Maybe we should go back to the original issue . . . that people feel like they're walking on eggshells around him. What does that mean?

STAFF MEMBER 2: He just gives you the feeling that he could explode at any minute.

MEDICAL DIRECTOR: Presumably, that's because we don't know him very well yet. You know what they say . . . if you're scared that a dog is going to bite you your most important task is to get to know the dog. Once you know the dog, you're a whole lot less worried about whether he's going to bite you. So Tyrone has been here 2 days. I know it's a little early, but what are our hypotheses about pathways at this point? I heard something about hyperactivity.

CHARGE NURSE: What I've been hearing is that he seems extremely irritable. In fact, he's telling people he feels like he's very on edge.

MEDICAL DIRECTOR: Do we have a medication history?

SOCIAL WORKER: The guidance counselor at his current school says the grandmother is very suspicious of psychiatrists, so she's been very reluctant to use medicine.

MEDICAL DIRECTOR: Besides him telling us that he's on edge, do we have any other suggestion of irritability?

STAFF MEMBER 3: I was on shift last night. Eddie bumped up against him accidentally, and I was sure Tyrone was going to lose it. He spun around and screamed, "You got a problem?" Luckily, Eddie's not the type to go toe-to-toe with people. Eddie kinda put his hands up and said, "Just an accident. Sorry." But Tyrone looked like he was ready to kill him.

CHARGE NURSE: This morning he couldn't find his toothbrush. He was sure someone stole it from him. It took me 10 minutes to reassure him that it probably wasn't stolen and that it was probably just misplaced. We finally found it.

STAFF PSYCHOLOGIST: Hmm. I don't know if that's irritability or cognitive distortions. Of course it could be both.

SOCIAL WORKER: I think that's cognitive distortions. The person at his school said Tyrone trusts no one. His grandmother trusts no one. He's actually made statements suggesting that he thinks people are out to get him.

STAFF PSYCHOLOGIST: So we've got two potential skill areas that we need more information about. I think we should let staff know that we're interested in their observations about those skills today. Given that people feel like they're walking on eggshells, it sounds like we need to be very aggressive in gathering information about Tyrone's thinking skills. Has he been interacting with the other kids since he was admitted?

CHARGE NURSE: He mostly keeps to himself. He seems more interested in talking with staff than with the other kids.

STAFF MEMBER 1: Forgive me, but I don't understand why his lagging skills matter so much. I mean, how is that going to help us keep him from going crazy on us?

STAFF PSYCHOLOGIST: Well, knowing about his lagging skills may help you predict what's going to set him off. But mostly it gives you information about what you're trying to do to keep him from exploding in the first place.

STAFF MEMBER 1: I still don't get it.

STAFF PSYCHOLOGIST: Well, let's say he's irritable. He could just be agitated that he's been placed on an inpatient unit again. He could be agitated about something that was going on in his life before he got admitted—like whatever caused him to try to strangle his grandmother. I think if one of those things is fueling his irritability, we'd want to put a lot of effort into trying to engage him so he'll start communicating with us. Of course, it could also be that he's chronically irritable. If that's the issue, we might consider medication, if the grandmother would allow it. Either way, at least he knows we're aware of his irritability and knows that he can communicate with us about it. So at least we're not the enemy . . . we understand. But if we're also dealing with cognitive distortions—people are out to get me, you can't trust anybody—then we've got more to work on with him than just irritability. Those thoughts could make it very hard for him to confide in us, so we'd want to be aware of their possible influence on how he interacts with us. I don't think we have enough information yet to know what we're working on. That's why we need to observe and gently inquire.

MEDICAL DIRECTOR: So let's translate that into what we want staff doing with Tyrone today and how we want people interacting with him. In other words, let's think about how we want people to further assess Tyrone's pathways today so we don't get bit by the dog.

CHARGE NURSE: I think we want to get a handle on what's going on with him when he starts getting upset. Is he thinking that people are out to get him or is he just irritable?

STAFF MEMBER 2: You mean, ask him what he's feeling?

STAFF PSYCHOLOGIST: I think we're interested in what he's feeling, if he's got the words to describe it. But I think we're mostly interested in what he's thinking, given the possibility of cognitive distortions.

STAFF MEMBER 2: What if he won't tell us? I mean, if he doesn't trust people, why would he tell us?

STAFF PSYCHOLOGIST: If he doesn't tell us, that could be good assessment information. Of course, we'd need to get a fix on whether he didn't want to tell us or didn't feel like he had the words to tell us. But from what I'm hearing, he seems pretty receptive to being heard.

STAFF MEMBER 2: What if he starts going nuts?

CHARGE NURSE: Then we'll do what we usually do: try to find out what his concern is and try to solve the problem that got him upset in the first place. I'm just saying it would be a lot better to get the information proatively rather than emergently.

Staff members in all therapeutic facilities have diverse opinions about the factors underlying residents' maladaptive behavior. We have observed that this divide can be particularly acute in facilities housing juvenile offenders. While data indicate that youth in such facilities have very much the same psychiatric issues as youth in other therapeutic settings, the fact that incarcerated youth have broken the law can cause some staff to be less sensitive to these issues and treat such youth like little criminals. Of course, it doesn't help matters that so many such facilities are referred to as "corrections" settings. We find that these youth have far greater need of *good therapy* than of being *corrected*.

STAFF PSYCHOLOGIST: I think it would be good if we talked about George today.

SECURITY OFFICER 1: That is one devious dude.

SOCIAL WORKER: I guess I don't see him as devious . . . just closed for business.

MILIEU STAFF MEMBER 1: What do you mean?

SOCIAL WORKER: Well, he's been here a long time . . . I've been trying to get to know him a long time . . . and he just gives you very little to go on.

SECURITY OFFICER 1: That's what I mean . . . he's devious.

STAFF PSYCHOLOGIST: What do you mean by devious?

SECURITY OFFICER 1: Look, he's here because he has a long history of assaults . . . he's hurt some people pretty bad. He's never expressed any remorse about that. In fact, I heard him bragging about it the other day. That's what I call devious. That boy is just a psychopath.

STAFF PSYCHOLOGIST: Well, I think it's easy to throw these terms around . . . devious, psychopathic . . . but I don't think it gets us any closer to understanding him or what he needs.

SECURITY OFFICER 2: Don't you think that there are some residents who are just criminals . . . and that's their only pathway?

STAFF PSYCHOLOGIST: I know that "criminal" isn't one of the items on the Pathways Inventory. That's why I think we need to be much more specific about what you mean.

SOCIAL WORKER: One of the things we know about him is that he has a substance use problem. And, if you're asking me what skill he's lacking, I'd say the number one skill he's lacking is empathy.

SECURITY OFFICER 1: That's what I'm talking about . . . the kid just has no feelings. He doesn't care about anyone but himself. Isn't that the definition of a psychopath?

STAFF PSYCHOLOGIST: I think that calling him a psychopath just makes it easy for us to write him off. I think we take pride on not writing kids off, no matter how difficult they are to reach. I don't see how calling him a psychopath helps us understand what skills he's lacking or help us know what we're trying to teach.

SECURITY OFFICER 1: But that's my point . . . some residents . . . I think a lot of 'em . . . *can't* be taught. That's why they're here.

SOCIAL WORKER: I'm not convinced that's the best way to understand George. In fact, I think it's possible that his not talking to us has less to do with being devious and more to do with him being scared that something he tells us could be used against him in his trial.

SECURITY OFFICER 2: Sounds pretty devious to me.

STAFF PSYCHOLOGIST: You know, it's interesting . . . if he's not talking to us because he's worried that something he tells us could be used against him in his trial . . . then doesn't that tell us he does care about something?

SECURITY OFFICER 1: Yeah, it tells me he cares about himself!

STAFF PSYCHOLOGIST: Well, we don't know if his apparent lack of caring about his victims is bravado . . . for the sake of the other residents . . . or how he really feels. What I'm saying is that a few minutes ago, we were hypothesizing that George doesn't care about anything . . . now we seem to be agreeing that he may well care very much about what happens to him in court.

SOCIAL WORKER: I think he's petrified that they're going to try him as an adult. I just wish he'd let us talk to him about that.

UNIT DIRECTOR: I think he's petrified, too. Occasionally he'll let it slip that he's worried about what's going to happen to him.

SECURITY OFFICER 2: So how come when he's talking about his victims he's got a smile on his face?

SOCIAL WORKER: If I've learned anything in this business, it's that facial expression and bravado often don't tell the tale. I don't think we want to base all our judgments about his character on his facial expression.

STAFF PSYCHOLOGIST: Question is, could we be using Plan B more effectively to get him to talk to us about what he's going through? Then at least we'd have a better idea about where he's coming from. In other words, what would we say to try to empathize with him?

SOCIAL WORKER: How about something like "I guess you must be worried that something you say to us could come up in your trial."

UNIT DIRECTOR: That probably summarizes it.

STAFF PSYCHOLOGIST: Then our concern would be that it's hard to help him if he doesn't feel like he can trust us.

UNIT DIRECTOR: He's going to say that he doesn't want our help.

SOCIAL WORKER: Maybe we shouldn't say we're trying to help him. Maybe we just want to know him a little better. What are we trying to do with him?

STAFF PSYCHOLOGIST: See, I think that our impression that he's a psychopath or devious has prevented us from thinking about the pathways! For all we know, he's not talking to us because he doesn't have the words!

SOCIAL WORKER: So maybe I need to be more direct with him and actually ask him if he knows why he's having so much trouble telling us what's going on. In all the time I've been working with him, I've never asked him that question!

UNIT DIRECTOR: Think he'll be honest with you if he knows the answer?

SOCIAL WORKER: I don't know. I do know that so long as we keep calling him a psychopath . . . so long as we don't focus on his pathways . . . we're not working on anything with him.

Of course, once pathways have been tentatively identified, the discussion turns to action plans for how and by whom the pathways are to be further assessed and ways in which the resident should be handled in certain circumstances. By "action plan," of course, we are referring primarily to the assessment information staff are trying to gather (Will the additional information we're hoping to obtain from the resident be gathered by the resident's individual therapist that day or through casual discussions with a milieu staff member?) and the triggers we are trying to address (What Proactive Plan B discussions do we need to have with the resident today? Which staff member is initiating what discussion?).

OTHER CHANGES

As staff members become increasingly comfortable with the CPS model, it sometimes becomes apparent that the very manner in which the unit is organized (scheduling, grouping, expectations, staffing patterns, mechanisms of communication, etc.) may actually be making it *more difficult* for staff members to observe, assess, collaboratively problem-solve, and teach. On one inpatient unit, for example, it became clear that a small number of residents was "messing up the milieu" for the remaining residents. Through discussion, it was agreed that these residents simply were not yet able to participate fully in the therapeutic program of the unit. Once this problem was identified, staff collaborated on generating solutions (here the CPS model applies to adult–adult interactions rather than merely adult–resident interactions). Through a process of staff brainstorming, it was agreed that the unit would be divided into two groups: those residents who were not yet ready to participate in most of the therapeutic activities of the unit nor able to respond to the same expectations as the other residents (therefore requiring a smaller resident–staff ratio) and those who were able to participate in therapeutic activities and adhere to most unit expectations (and required the supervision of fewer staff members). Once those in the former group were well assessed and stabilized, they were integrated into the latter group.

Future discussions on the same unit focused on the daily schedule. Staff came to feel that the sheer number of therapy groups in which residents were expected to participate was extreme, and that enforcing attendance at groups accounted for many unnecessary explosive episodes. It was agreed that the number of daily therapy groups should be reduced and expectations for attendance individualized.

STAFF MEMBER 1: So we're not making kids go to therapy group anymore?

MEDICAL DIRECTOR: Making them go? No. Expecting them to go? Yes.

STAFF MEMBER 1: So what do I do if Jamal won't go to therapy group?

STAFF MEMBER 2: Ask him what's up. After you get his concern on the table, get yours on the table. Then solve the problem in a way that addresses both concerns. But let's not wait until he's balking at going to group before we try Plan B . . . we need to have that conversation with him way before he's balking at going to group.

Other discussions centered on the highly variable mix of residents on the unit; during some days and weeks the mix was particularly challenging, and this required alterations in staffing assignments and expectations. Ultimately, staff found that a daily assessment of unit needs was necessary and that a highly flexible approach to the organization and schedule of the unit was ideal. CPS helps staff feel that they are important, empowered, and valued members of a problem-solving team. The goal is not to ensure that each resident, regardless of need, fit into a "round hole," but to create a therapeutic environment that can be readily adapted to any variety of "square pegs." The ideal structure is one that is able to accommodate the population of residents placed on the unit at any given time.

For example, on one child inpatient unit, a situational analysis suggested that a particular resident was most explosive at bedtime when he refused to sleep in his room alone. Exploration of his concerns through a Proactive Plan B discussion led to the understanding that his trauma history made him frightened of intruders in his room at night. With flexibility being the rule and not the exception, staff and the resident together identified a place to sleep that would be comfortable for him (in this case, on a mattress outside the nurse's station). In another case, a child with severe obsessive–compulsive symptoms frequently exploded at the thought of having to use the common bathrooms. Through a Proactive Plan B discussion, staff and the resident dedicated a particular sink and toilet to this child for the first few days after his admission in order to help stabilize him and assess what other pathways, if any, were contributing to his oppositional and aggressive behavior. Of course, some staff may initially have difficulty adapting to the "fair does not mean equal" principle, especially if they've become accustomed to achieving "consistency" through a level system. But "good care" doesn't look the same for every resident because every resident has different needs.

On an adolescent inpatient unit, lively discussions centered on whether some residents should be permitted to smoke. The situational analysis had established that many explosive episodes were occurring when nicotine-addicted residents were denied smoking privileges (unit policy prohibited all smoking), thereby completely eclipsing the issues that had landed the resident on the inpatient unit in the first place. Again, these discussions focused on staff concerns about giving residents the wrong message ("What, we're going to tell them that smoking is OK?"). Ultimately, staff came to the consensus that, since smoking was never the issue that precipitated inpatient admissions in the first place, having rigid restrictions on smoking was a red herring, and new policies for smoking were enacted. Similar fascinating and energetic discussions took place as regards physical contact between residents. When is a hug or a pat romantic versus supportive? Are there circumstances under which it is OK for residents to hold hands? Are there some residents who should not touch or be touched? Ultimately, the unit created policies that took staff concerns and the needs of individual residents into account.

There are many other changes to existing policies, procedures, and structures that may occur once a staff begins to question existing practices. For example, one possible outgrowth of implementing CPS in a restrictive facility may be changes to policies regarding visitation. In one particular setting, approximately 3 months after the initiation of CPS, the unit adopted an open visitation policy in which parents were permitted access to the unit at any time, including overnight. There were many good reasons to make this change, foremost among them that it was difficult to engage some working parents because they were unable to visit the unit during normal visiting hours and that staff wanted to encourage parents and other caretakers to observe Plan B in action on the unit. The open-door policy also helped enhance the comfort level among highly anxious children. On the same unit, special attention was also paid to the scheduling of staff to ensure that each shift comprised some staff members who were more adept at the new model of care.

As noted above, another crucial change necessitated by implementation of CPS is to improve staff communication. Clearly, the CPS model requires far greater communication between staff and shifts than mere transfer of information regarding checks (i.e., how much time can elapse before staff must visually ensure that a resident is safe), diagnosis, medication regimen, and level. While different settings have adopted different strategies along these lines, we have developed a form called the Individualized Cognitive Challenges Plan (ICCP) to ensure that information gleaned about a resident in rounds or on a given shift can be communicated to other staff members in an efficient manner (see Figure 8.1). The ICCP also indicates whether a resident is expected to participate in various unit activities and communicates the specific issues to be discussed with each resident with Plan B during upcoming shifts.

RESEARCH

The effectiveness of the CPS model in restrictive facilities has been documented in one study (Greene, Ablon, Hassuk, Regan, Markey, & Goring, in press), with elimination of chemical, physical, and mechanical restraint and locked-door seclusion and rates of staff and patient injuries as the primary out-come variables. Current practice parameters mandate that R/S procedures are indicated only to prevent dangerous behavior to self or others and to prevent disorganization or serious disruption of the treatment program, and only when less restrictive options have failed or are impractical (American Academy of Child and Adolescent Psychiatry, 2002). Practice parameters further mandate that seclusion or restraint not be used as punishment for patients, for the conve-nience of the program, or to compensate for inadequate staffing patterns (American Academy of Child and Adolescent Psychiatry, 2002). Consistent with the CPS model, it has been argued that altering the manner by which lim-its are set on an inpatient unit may be particularly important to reducing R/S procedures, and there is evidence indicating that some type of redirection or limit setting by staff precipitates most assaults by patients (Ryan, Hart, Messick, Aaron, & Burnette, 2004).

The study took place on a 13-bed, locked unit, admitting children be-tween the ages of 4 and 14 years. The average length of stay on the unit was 14 days. Approximately 80% of the children admitted to the unit have significant trauma histories, and 95% are admitted for severe out-of-control behavior at home or at school. The most common diagnoses are oppositional defiant disor-der, post-traumatic stress disorder, mood disorders, anxiety disorders, perva-sive developmental disorders, and psychotic disorders. Many of the children have suffered major losses in their lives as a result of the death, incarceration, or absence of a parent or caregiver, which has resulted in placements in kin-ship, foster, or adoptive homes or in residential facilities.

Pretraining was defined as the 3–9 months preceding implementation of CPS. The modifications/training phase occurred during the subsequent 12 months, beginning with a 6-month period in which there was a change in unit leadership (nursing manager and medical director), active questioning of unit policies and procedures (including a focus on the true necessity of R/S procedures), and preparation for implementation of the CPS model (pri-marily involving orientation of the new unit leadership), followed by a 6-month period in which staff were trained in the CPS model, including inten-sive supervision of milieu staff. Follow-up data were collected during the 15 months of ongoing implementation subsequent to the active training phase. Thirty-four staff members from the unit participated in CPS training (10 males and 24 females). The staff represented diverse roles on the unit, in-cluding 10 nurses, three social workers, 13 milieu counselors, one activities counselor, one teacher, one psychologist, one physician, two student train-ees, and two administrative assistants. One hundred children (74 males and 26 females, mean age = 9.14 years) were admitted to the unit during the ac-tive training of milieu staff. Training of milieu staff involved an initial 3-hour

Name of Child:

Date:

I. History/Psychosocial Stressors:

II. Pathways *Use this section to specify the lagging thinking skills that are **currently** being targeted for intervention. (Use the Pathways Inventory to document the full array of lacking thinking skills that apply to this individual):*

___ self-injurious behavior	___ assaultive to others	___ suicidal intent
___ victim of physical abuse	___ victim of emotional abuse	___ sexual abuse
		___ placement in residential care
___ placed in foster care	___ adopted	___ eating disorder
___ incarceration	___ inpatient admissions	___ school suspension, expulsion
___ substance abuse	___ learning disabilities	
___ surrogate parents	___ parent mental illness	___ parent incarceration

III. Triggers *Use this section to specify the events/situations that are currently being targeted for intervention. (Use the Pathways Inventory to document the full range of triggers that routinely precipitate challenging behavior):*

IV. Action Plan:

1) **PLAN B CONVERSATION PENDING** *Use this section to specify a problem (trigger) or lagging skill (pathway) that requires a Plan B discussion with the resident or student, and specify the staff member assigned to initiate this discussion:*

2) **PLAN B SOLUTION AGREED UPON** *Use this section to specify the solution or plan mutually agreed upon in a Plan B discussion with the resident or student so that other staff are aware of the how a specific problem is being handled or lagging thinking skill being addressed:*

3) **ACCOMMODATE/ADAPT** *Use this section to specify any expectations that are being eliminated (handled with Plan C) or adapted for this resident or student:*

FIGURE 8.1. Collaborative Problem Solving. Individualized Cognitive Challenges Plan.

orientation for all staff, followed by 4 hours of weekly supervision (two 2-hour sessions).

Many changes in the culture of the unit occurred as a by-product of the training and supervision in the CPS model. For example, the number of therapy groups in which patients were expected to participate was reduced as staff came to the realization that enforcing attendance at such groups accounted for many unnecessary explosive outbursts. Rather than having all patients together on the milieu at all times, staff began working with children in smaller groups, with particular attention to the grouping of children whom staff believed were not yet able to participate fully in unit activities (this assessment was made on a daily basis). Further, the structure of the unit became more flexible in an attempt to be responsive to the "mix" of patients on the unit at any given time. A concerted attempt was made by supervisors to identify and provide additional counseling to staff who were having difficulty adapting to the new model of care and their new roles as observers, teachers, and problem solvers. Nonetheless, the staff attrition rate during active training was approximately 30%. Moreover, special attention was paid to the scheduling of staff to ensure that each shift was comprised of some staff members who were more adept at the new model of care. Approximately 3 months after the initiation of the active implementation phase, the unit adopted an open visiting policy in which parents were permitted access to the unit at any time (including overnight). Finally, initiation of CPS required significant support from top hospital administrators and attention to union issues.

To assess whether the severity of impairment of children admitted to the unit remained constant during the modifications/training phase, the ODD Rating Scale (ODDRS) was completed by staff three times daily for each child on the unit at any given time. The ODDRS has been used in previous studies (e.g., Greene et al., 2004) to assess oppositional and aggressive behavior in children. This measure consists of the DSM-IV diagnostic criteria for oppositional defiant disorder rated on a Likert scale. ODDRS scores were unchanged over time, suggesting that unit acuity remained constant during active training.

Data regarding restraint and seclusion were collected during the 9 months preceding active training; data regarding staff and patient injuries were collected during the 3 months preceding active training. Data for both outcomes variables were also collected during the 12-month modifications/training phase and for the 15-month follow-up phase, during which implementation of CPS and other modifications were ongoing.

Results showed a significant decrease in rates of restraint and seclusion between the pretraining and follow-up phases. During the 9 months preceding the modifications/training phase, a total of 281 restraints were utilized. By contrast, one restraint was utilized in the 15 months of ongoing implementation following training.

Data regarding rates of physical holds under 5 minutes were not collected during the first two phases of the study, but were collected later in the ongoing implementation phase. These data show that physical holds under 5 minutes were dramatically reduced on the unit over time as well.

Results also revealed a significant decrease in staff and patient injuries between the pretraining and follow-up phases. During the pretraining phase there was an average of 10.75 staff and patient injuries per month; during the follow-up phase, the unit averaged 3.29 injuries per month.

While the above study certainly possesses ecological validity, there are a variety of limitations in its research design imposed by the realities of conducting such real-world research. It was not possible to control for the many changes that occurred on the inpatient unit as a by-product of CPS training. Thus, it is not possible to parse out those changes principally accounting for the positive changes in unit culture. On a related note, in a "purer" research design we might have tracked rates of restraint and seclusion initiated by specific staff members. Recall that the staff attrition rate during the active implementation phase was approximately 30% (of course, staff attrition prior to implementation was also quite high). The degree to which the departed staff members were those largely responsible for rates of restraint and seclusion prior to implementation of the model is unknown. While the above study took place on a *child* inpatient unit, similar results have been achieved on an *adolescent* unit as well and are currently well underway in multiple juvenile detention and residential facilities.

Chapter 9

Last Call

Chapters 1 through 8 provided a very detailed overview of the CPS model. And yet, while we've been quite specific in delineating many of the basic facets of the model and answered many of the common questions we encounter, it's quite common for many clinicians to have lingering questions and concerns. And parents, teachers, and other caregivers often have many of the same questions. So let's kill two birds with one stone: in answering your questions, we'll also help you answer theirs.

In Chapter 1, you discussed Baumrind's categories of parenting styles. Which category does Plan B fall into?
None of them. It certainly doesn't fall into either the "permissive" or "authoritarian" categories. While it comes closest to the "authoritative" category, recall that authoritative parents who are warm and nurturing are still imposing limits, demands, and controls and the types of limits, demands, and controls Baumrind envisioned bear greater resemblance to Plan A than Plan B.

So is CPS a parent-centered or child-centered model?
Neither. And both.

We don't live in a Plan B world. We live in a Plan A world. So while Plan B may help adults pursue expectations without causing oppositional episodes, adults in the real world aren't likely to pursue expectations that way. Aren't we setting the kid up for a fall?

First, we're not so sure we live in a Plan A world. We like to ask people to ponder the following question: Which skill is more important to train to a child with respect to his long-term development, blind adherence to authority (as trained with Plan A) or learning how to work things out with people in a mutually satisfactory manner (as trained by Plan B)? We pick door number two. We actually think that blind adherence to authority is not a skill that we call upon very often and dangerous in a democratic society that depends on people being able to think things through, problem-solve, and make decisions that take different perspectives into account. And if people ask, "What if he has a Plan A boss someday?" our response is, "A Plan A boss is a problem to be solved. That skill is taught with Plan B."

It's important to remain focused on the learning disability conceptualization of oppositional behavior. If a child has a reading disability, we don't throw the *Encyclopaedia Britannica* at him and say "Read!" in anticipation of him needing to read the *Encyclopaedia Brittanica* in the real world. We train the lacking skill in increments he can handle. The concept is the same here. You don't help a child who doesn't have a Plan A brain by throwing him into the Plan A frying pan. First you identify his lacking cognitive skills. Then you make sure everyone who comes into contact with the child knows about them. Then you set the stage for each of them to start training those lacking skills. Yes, this sometimes requires several visits to the child's school, if oppositional episodes are occurring there. It sometimes means making sure that grandparents come to your sessions if they are important caretakers and still invested in Plan A. No, this is not easy, and it can be labor-intensive. But fixing the problem is always less labor-intensive than not fixing the problem.

We were all raised with Plan A and turned out fine, right? Why change the way we've always done things?

It depends what you mean by "fine." We wonder if teaching a child that his concerns are secondary to adult concerns, that adults have no faith in his ability to solve problems, and that adults are the only people who are truly capable of coming up with good solutions to problems is really the best way to go about setting the stage for a healthy adulthood. We think these lessons have the potential to set the stage for later relationship problems and other forms of psychopathology. And we don't want to forget about the many adults who were raised with Plan A and currently reside in corrections facilities.

But it's important for kids to respect authority, yes?

Yes, of course . . . but we don't think the respect should be automatic. Before kids can respect authority adults must behave in ways that engender respect. Kids don't respect adults who continue to apply Plan A to problems that Plan A hasn't fixed. Kids do respect adults who have reasonable expectations, listen to their concerns, treat them with mutual respect, and work toward finding mutually satisfactory solutions.

What do you say when parents or teachers want to know how to tell the difference between when a child's behavior is manipulative and when it is driven by a poor response to frustration?

We don't know anyone who can reliably distinguish between the two patterns. Earlier we noted that the children with whom we work typically lack the requisite skills (forethought, planning, impulse control, organization) for competent manipulation. While we understand that children sometimes behave in a difficult fashion in hopes of convincing an adult to give in, we also know that this is not the only explanation for children's social, emotional, and behavioral challenges.

The data presented in Chapter 1 tell the tale: oppositional behavior almost always occurs concurrently with other psychiatric conditions. While we are careful in making assumptions about directionality, we think it's likely that executive deficits contribute to the development of oppositional behavior rather than the reverse. We think it's likely that language deficits contribute to the development of oppositional behavior rather than the reverse. And we think that concrete, black-and-white thinking is likely to contribute to oppositional behavior rather than the reverse. We think assessment of these deficits should begin the instant a child begins to demonstrate chronic difficulties handling frustration and responding to the world in an adaptive, flexible manner (rather than only after conventional behavior management strategies have failed).

Moreover, we see no risk in treating even children who are believed to be truly manipulative through Plan B (remember, a mutually satisfactory solution requires that both parties' concerns be addressed). Indeed, we think manipulation can best be conceived as a very indirect way to solve a problem, and as a byproduct of the direct route to problem solving having been blocked. Plan B is a direct route to problem solving and eliminates the need for manipulation.

How do you respond when adults ask if the CPS model says there should be no consequences for anything?

By definition, a *consequence* is an event that occurs after the fact. So consequences—especially the natural variety—are inescapable (the child who lacks social skills has no friends; the child who doesn't do his homework receives a failing grade). Thus, this question usually refers to *formal* consequences. For the record, we think formal consequences are wonderful, but only when they are effective. We are significantly less enthusiastic about formal consequences when they are ineffective. We think consequences are effective at two things: (1) teaching a child basic lessons—for example, don't hit, don't swear, don't explode (of course, we would only teach these lessons if we were convinced that a child was unaware of them); and (2) giving a child the incentive to behave adaptively (assuming, of course, that the child is not motivated already). Since every child we've worked with was already familiar with the basic lessons and since we believe children are already motivated to behave adaptively (secondary gain is, we believe, greatly overrated as an explanation for why a child would choose to endure repeated punishment), we have difficulty appreciating the role consequences might play in the treatment of an explosive kid. We don't think it makes sense to use consequences just because consequences are the only tools in one's toolbox.

Can CPS be implemented in tandem with contingency management procedures? In other words, can the two models be used together? Is it a good idea to reward a child for using Plan B?

In research the two models have been combined, and with good results. In a series of studies, Alan Kazdin and colleagues (1987, 1992) examined the relative and combined effects of a family problem-solving model (not CPS, but something similar) and a consequence-based, contingency management model in youth with conduct problems. The combined treatment was more effective than either of the two models alone, though differences that emerged between the two single treatments tended to favor the problem-solving model (we found the same pattern in our own initial study of the effectiveness of CPS, described below).

However, as a matter of practice, we generally stay away from combining the two models. Because children are typically not involved in the development of their own contingency management programs, are not given the option to go to time-out, and are not engaged in discussions about suitable consequences for their actions, these procedures are distinctly Plan A. Thus, when a child doesn't receive the reward he was hoping for, is sent or escorted to time-out, or receives a punishment, the likelihood of an explosive episode is greatly increased. We think the same problem that caused the child to lose the reward, receive the time-out, or be punished can just as easily be resolved with Plan B without the risk of an explosive episode (while simultaneously teaching lacking cognitive skills). It's also worth pondering whether either of the two things consequences do well—teaching basic lessons and motivating (see above)—are really coming into play. If not, we see no reason to add a contingency management component. Moreover, because the two models conceptualize children's difficulties differently and therefore lead to very different "action plans," we find that combining the two models can be very confusing to adults. And confused adults tend to head for familiar ground (Plan A). Should a child be rewarded for participating in Plan B? We think successfully executed Plan B—solving the problem, communicating, enhancing the adult–child relationship—is far more rewarding than any extrinsic motivator.

My background is in learning theory, and the CPS model is making me a little uneasy. You seem to be saying that explosive episodes do not cause a child to learn that adults will capitulate to his or her wishes. Does this mean that you think no learning is occurring? How can this be?
      Learning is continuous and inexorable. In its focus on antecedent events, cognition, and situational specificity, learning theory (as in social learning theory) is the central theoretical underpinning of the CPS model. What we reject is the automatic assumption that a child has learned that explosive episodes are an effective means of seeking attention or coercing adults into capitulating. Thus, we also reject the automatic premise that what a child needs to be taught is that his explosive episodes will not attract attention (adults typically teach this lesson by withdrawing reinforcement, otherwise known as ignoring or time-out) and that adults will not even discuss the concerns that caused the child to become frustrated in the first place (thereby eliminating the possibility of capitulation). In actuality, there are many other things a child could have learned from his or her repeated explosive episodes. He might have learned that when he becomes frustrated, his adult interaction partners often become frustrated as well, and that this compounds his initial frustration. He might also have learned that his adult interaction partners become highly inflexible and rigid themselves when he becomes frustrated, and aren't exactly sure how to proceed in a manner that will effectively reduce his frustration. He most certainly has learned that punishment is often the end result of these episodes, and that the punishment doesn't seem to be making things any better.

It follows that there are many other things a child could be taught; for example, that adults are able to respond to his frustration in a manner that reduces agitation, resolves frustrations in a mutually satisfactory manner, teaches lacking thinking skills, and makes things better.

But if a child exhibits the desired behavior every once in a while, doesn't that mean that he's capable of behaving correctly and that lack of motivation is the problem?

The two authors of this book are highly motivated to sink 30-foot jump shots on the basketball court all the time, but only accomplish the feat every so often. Solving the problem would require either significant practice/ instruction or adjusted expectations. Adding incentives would not be likely to improve motivation . . . authors do well if they can, too.

What are the most common problems you see in therapists trying to implement this model?

We find that, early on, many therapists attempting to implement CPS don't feel completely comfortable with the pathways and continue to describe children's difficulties using diagnoses. Remember, a diagnosis gives no information about the specific thinking skills a given child may be lacking, and therefore does not point therapy in a direction as it relates to what skills are to be trained. Clinicians new to this approach are often too eager to introduce the plans—usually because they want to be responsive to the family's level of distress but also because they are eager to have some practical tools to offer—and therefore completely bypass the pathways. But there is a danger in introducing the plans before the parents have been convinced of the existence of cognitive skills deficits and signed on to their new role. So long as a parent still believes that a child is willfully misbehaving, that same parent will have no rationale for the use of Plan B. Finally, we find that many therapists have been trained to be good and empathic listeners and are therefore reluctant to be as directive in therapy as the CPS model demands.

How does CPS differ from anger management programs?

In placing primary emphasis on training children to manage their anger, many existing programs are quite explicit in targeting an "identified patient" (the child) and lose sight of the transactional nature of the child's interactions with the world. Moreover, such training typically takes place outside of the contexts (e.g., in a therapist's office or a guidance counselor's office) in which the child is having difficulty. The child is then sent back into the "real world," armed with new skills so as to be the primary agent of change. In the CPS model, training involves all relevant interaction partners—in other words, there is no identified patient. Thus, the training takes place in the environments where the child is having the greatest difficulty and everyone learns the skills.

Are there data regarding the effectiveness of the CPS model in outpatient settings?

The first controlled treatment outcome study examining the effectiveness of CPS has been published (Greene, Ablon, Monuteaux, et al., 2004). The study involved 50 children between the ages of 4 and 12 years meeting diagnostic criteria for oppositional defiant disorder (ODD) who were randomly assigned (using a 3:2 randomization scheme) to CPS or parent training (PT). Three children (two in the CPS condition and one in the PT condition) did not complete treatment. Thus, 28 children completed treatment in the CPS condition, 19 in the PT condition. All children were clinically referred (to an outpatient mental health clinic specializing in the treatment of disruptive behavior disorders at a university teaching hospital); all met full diagnostic criteria for ODD; none met full diagnostic criteria for CD at the time of enrollment in the study (but many had subthreshold features of CD). All children also had at least subthreshold features of either juvenile bipolar disorder or major depression (defined as more than half of the symptoms needed to meet criteria for the diagnosis). Children were ineligible to participate if they had an estimated Full Scale IQ below 80 or were actively suicidal or homicidal on entry into the study. The final sample included five children of minority ethnicity (4 African American and 1 Asian American). Eighty-seven percent (PT, $n = 16$; CPS, $n = 25$) of the children who completed treatment were available for follow-up assessment at 4 months post treatment.

Those families assigned to the PT condition received Barkley's (1997b) 10-week behavior management program. This treatment program is manualized, with specified weekly session content. Families in this treatment condition received 10 weeks of treatment, as prescribed by the treatment manual. Treatment sessions in this condition were attended primarily by parents, with identified children included as indicated by the training manual. The remaining families were assigned to the CPS condition. The range of treatment sessions in the CPS condition was 7–16 weeks, and the mean length of treatment in this condition was 11 weeks. Treatment sessions in this condition were attended primarily by parents, with identified children included at the discretion of the therapist.

All clinicians were experienced PhD-level clinical psychologists. Two clinicians delivered PT; four different clinicians delivered CPS. Therapists in the PT condition identified behavior therapy as their primary therapeutic modality and had considerable experience in providing PT; therapists in the CPS condition identified cognitive-behavioral therapy as their primary therapeutic orientation. Therapists in both treatment modalities received weekly supervision from the principal investigator (PI) to ensure adherence to treatment manuals. While the PI's supervision of both treatment conditions represented a potential methodological problem (i.e., possible disparate levels of expertise in the two treatments or greater investment in one of the two conditions), having different supervisors for the two groups of therapists might have simply pitted one supervisor's skill against another's. The adherence/integrity data reported below help alleviate concerns along these lines.

No medication was prescribed or administered as a component of either treatment condition. However, to enhance the ecological validity of the study (and taking into account the volatility and high level of aggressiveness of the population of children under study), children were permitted to remain on existing pharmacological regimens upon entry into the study, and the study did not mandate that medication regimens remain unaltered during active treatment. Parents provided information about each child's medication regimens on a weekly basis to document initial regimen at the commencement of active treatment and any changes (removing or adding medications or switching from one medication to another within the same class of medications) that occurred during treatment.

The Kiddie-SADS—Epidemiologic Version (K-SADS-E; Orvaschel, 1994) was used to assess children's diagnostic status prior to enrollment in the active treatment phase of the study. Interviewers administering the K-SADS-E also assigned a DSM-IV Global Assessment of Functioning (GAF) score to each child based on information obtained in the diagnostic interview. The GAF score summarizes a child's global functioning and psychopathology using a scale ranging from 1 (worst) to 90 (best). Socioeconomic status was determined using the Hollingshead (1975) four-factor scale. Using methods described by Sattler (1988), cognitive ability was estimated using age-corrected scaled scores in the Block Design and Vocabulary subtests from the Wechsler Intelligence Scale for Children—Revised (WISC-R; Wechsler, 1974).

All therapy sessions were audiotaped to assess treatment integrity. A rater unaware of the nature of the two treatment conditions (and therefore also unaware of the treatment being provided by specific therapists) listened to 20% of the tapes (randomly selected, with equal proportions of the two treatment conditions) and rated the degree to which various content consistent with the two treatment approaches was present during each session, using a treatment adherence scale developed for this study.

The Parent–Child Relationship Inventory (PCRI; Gerard, 1994) was completed by parents at pretreatment and posttreatment, and was used to assess the general quality of parent–child interactions. The Parenting Stress Index (PSI; Abidin, 1995) was completed by parents at pretreatment and posttreatment. The ODD Rating Scale (ODDRS) is an instrument listing the DSM-IV diagnostic criteria for ODD, rated for frequency and severity on a 5-point Likert scale (1 = false/never, 5 = always true/very often). A Clinical Global Impression instrument (CGI; National Institute of Mental Health, 1985) was completed by the therapist at posttreatment and by parents at 4-month follow-up. The CGI includes, on a 7-point Likert scale, a rating of the degree to which the child's behavior has improved since the beginning of treatment (ranging from "very much improved" to "very much worse").

For the majority of outcomes, we used generalized estimating equation models, modeling outcomes as a function of treatment group (CPS or PT), time (pretreatment, posttreatment, and, where applicable, 4-month follow-up), and their interaction. The statistical significance of each covariate in these regression models was determined by Wald's test. To assess group differences on the CGI at posttreatment and follow-up, regression analyses were used. Effect sizes (see Cohen, 1988) were calculated using d = mean of group 1 minus mean of group 2 divided by the pooled standard deviation, and were categorized as small ($d = 0.2$), moderate ($d = 0.5$) and large ($d = 0.8$). All relevant analyses were two-tailed; statistical significance was defined at the .05 level. Because data from fathers was frequently incomplete, data from parent ratings reported below refers to mothers' ratings.

At pretreatment, there were no significant differences between the two treatment groups in any demographic variables, past or current GAF scores, or rates of diagnostic comorbidity. Nor did the two groups differ significantly (based on generalized estimating equation models) on any measures of treatment outcome. There were also no significant differences between the two treatment groups in rates of children who were receiving psychotropic medication at pretreatment or at posttreatment. However, children in the CPS condition had significantly more adjustments to their medication regimens during active treatment compared to children in the PT condition. Further analyses showed that the vast majority of the children in both conditions had two or fewer changes to medication regimen during active treatment (PT = 100%, CPS = 71.4%), and that the number of changes in the CPS condition was inflated by eight subjects who had three or more medication changes during active treatment. Nonetheless, this difference between the two treatment groups was presumably also due to the presence of a medication education module in the CPS condition. While it can be argued that controlling for medication changes would constitute a premature dismantling of the CPS treatment modules, we accounted for differences in medication changes by running analyses comparing treatment outcomes in three separate ways: (1) including medication changes as a covariate; (2) not including medication changes as a covariate; and (3) not including medication changes as a covariate but removing the eight subjects in the CPS condition with three or more medication changes. Our findings did not differ across these three methodologies. However, because we wanted to ensure that our findings were not confounded by differences in medication changes between the two groups, results reported below are those in which the medication changes variable was included as a covariate, where applicable.

Duration of treatment was constant in the PT condition but variable in the CPS condition. To protect against the potential confounds this presented, we assessed the degree to which treatment duration was a significant predictor of outcome for all outcome variables; it was not. Our data indicated that the PT condition was characterized largely by PT-specific interventions with very little inclusion of content relevant to CPS, and that CPS was characterized exclusively by CPS-specific interventions with no inclusion of content relevant to PT.

On the ODDRS, the CPS condition produced significant improvement from pretreatment to posttreatment and from pretreatment to 4-month follow-up. Time by group interactions from pretreatment to posttreatment and from pretreatment to 4-month follow-up were nonsignificant. The ODDRS was also used to calculate effect sizes for both treatment conditions. Large effect sizes were found for both CPS (1.19) and PT (0.80) from pretreatment to posttreatment. From pretreatment to 4-month follow-up, a large effect size was found for CPS (1.19) and a moderate effect size for PT (0.48).

On the Total Score of the PSI, the CPS condition produced significant improvement from pretreatment to posttreatment. The time by group interaction was nonsignificant. Subsequent examination of PSI subscales showed that the CPS condition produced significant improvement in one parent domain (competence) and three child domains (distractibility/hyperactivity, adaptability, and reinforces parent). The CPS condition also produced borderline significant improvement in the mood domain. The time by group interaction was not significant on any subscale. Medication changes were not a significant predictor on any subscales of the PSI with the exception of the mood subscale.

On the PCRI, the CPS condition produced significant improvement on both the limit-setting subscale and the communication subscale. There was a borderline significant time by group interaction on the autonomy subscale, with children in the PT condition evidencing deterioration and children in the CPS condition evidencing improvement, from pretreatment to post-treatment. Medication changes were not a significant predictor on any sub-scales of the PCRI.

We next examined ratings of the two treatment conditions on the therapist-completed (at posttreatment) and parent-completed (at 4-month follow-up) CGI, entering treatment group and changes in medication regi-men as predictors in regression models. Treatment group emerged as a signifi-cant predictor at posttreatment and at 4-month follow-up, with the behavior of children in the CPS condition rated as having improved to a significantly greater degree as compared to children in the PT condition.

We identified children who evidenced an "excellent response to treat-ment" as those whose behavior was, at posttreatment (rated by therapists) and at 4-month follow-up (rated by mothers) as "very much improved" or "much improved" on the CGI. We used logistic regression models, entering treat-ment group and medication changes as predictors. At 4-month follow-up, treatment group was a significant predictor of excellent response to treat-ment; 80% of children in the CPS condition evidenced an excellent response to treatment at this data point, as compared with 44% of those in the PT condition.

Because normative data for the ODDRS are not available, we defined clinical significance as an improvement of 25% or greater in ODD-related behaviors (as measured by the ODDRS) between pretreatment and post-treatment and between pretreatment and 4-month follow-up (using meth-ods for defining clinical significance articulated by Jacobson and Truax [1991]). No significant differences were found between the two groups in rates of children evidencing clinically significant change. At posttreatment 46% of children in the CPS condition evidenced clinically significant im-provement, as compared with 37% of those in the PT condition. At 4-month follow-up, 60% ($n = 15/25$) of children in the CPS condition evidenced clini-cally significant improvement, as compared with 37% ($n = 6/16$) of those in the PT condition.

Several strengths of this study are noteworthy, including a clinically re-ferred, highly comorbid sample; random assignment to treatment condition; adherence testing; use of a well-established comparison treatment; and col-lection of follow-up data 4 months posttreatment (see Chambless et al., 1996).

One particular aspect of this study is worthy of further discussion. While the number of children beginning and ending the study on medication did not significantly differ between the two groups, children in the CPS condition had a significantly greater number of changes in their medication regimens compared to children in the PT condition, presumably due to the medication education module of the CPS approach. This module is included in the CPS model because some of the factors contributing to the development of ODD may be well addressed by pharmacotherapy.

Another design aspect of this study is also worthy of mention. The CPS condition, while manualized, did not involve application of circumscribed treatment content in specific sessions. Rather, in keeping with calls for greater "matching" of treatment ingredients to the needs of individual children and their families (Greene & Ablon, 2001) and greater flexibility in the application of manualized treatments (e.g., Kendall, Chu, Gifford, Hayes, & Nautu, 1998), therapists providing CPS determined session content based on their assessment of the clinical needs of each child and family from week to week, choosing from six treatment modules. Moreover, treatment duration was not circumscribed, although a limit of 16 sessions per child and family was imposed. We believe this high level of individualization enhances the ecological validity of the CPS model. Indeed, given the complex and heterogeneous parent and child characteristics thought to contribute to the development of ODD, individualization of treatment is viewed as indispensable. In addition, this flexibility may improve treatment compliance and enhance the transportability of this treatment approach (Kendall & Southam-Gerow, 1995). However, while it is likely that specific ingredients of the CPS model contributed to the treatment gains shown by participants in this condition, it is possible that these gains were also a reflection of the emphasis on individualized treatment. Along these lines, it is also possible that differences between groups were based not on discrepant improvement but rather differential satisfaction with the format of the CPS model.

While there is an obvious need for replication of the above findings in different sites and with larger samples, the data provide support for the notion that the CPS model has positive effects on more global domains of functioning in explosive/noncompliant youth and their parents, including reduced parenting stress, enhanced parent–child interactions, and reduced oppositional behavior. Research on more specific domains of functioning—specifically, the degree to which the skills-training component of the CPS model produced verifiable improvements in the cognitive skills being addressed via Plan B—was not the goal of the above study and therefore awaits examination.

Are there children with whom the CPS model will not work? For example, Plan B sounds like it requires some pretty intensive verbal give-and-take. Can children who are nonverbal be trained to do Plan B?

The above study suggests that there are some families who do not have an excellent response to the CPS model. However, given the relatively small sample, we don't have a great sense yet as to the types of families, parents, or children who might not respond optimally. We do hope to study this in a much larger sample (pending funding).

We do believe that for a child to participate in Plan B he must have the linguistic skills of a 3-year-old. As you read in Chapter 6, if a child is below this level we often find that we must train some basic linguistic skills (e.g., a rudimentary feeling vocabulary, a vocabulary for expressing basic needs and frustrations) or use pictures to participate in Plan B. We are often asked if very young children can participate in Plan B discussions. At the least, Plan B can be verbally modeled for very young children, whose receptive skills typically develop in advance of their expressive skills. But we don't find age to be the crucial variable, since we work with many 3-year-olds whose problem-solving skills are superior to those of many of the 17-year-olds with whom we work!

Chapter 10

Epilogue

Beyond Explosive Kids

We have come a long way. We began by suggesting that there is a tremendous need for creative, effective alternative psychosocial treatments for oppositional, defiant, aggressive children and adolescents and their parents, teachers, and other adult caretakers. Next, we articulated a cognitive framework for understanding their difficulties and identifying specific cognitive skills that often need to be trained. Then we described a simple framework for helping adults categorize the myriad ways in which problems or unmet expectations can be approached. We then provided considerable detail on the ins and outs of implementing Plan B—Collaborative Problem Solving—in families, schools, and therapeutic/restrictive facilities, and how to handle many of the difficulties that often arise as adults and children try to master Plan B. Along the way, we tried to answer many of the common questions we hear about the CPS model from mental health clinicians and those to whom they provide guidance. The CPS approach has evolved over the past 10 or so years, and this book is the most current representation of the model. But the model is a work in progress. We anticipate (with some excitement) that further refinement of the model is inevitable as we continue to receive feedback and discover ways to make the model more digestible and easier to implement.

Let us close by underscoring that we firmly believe that the CPS model can be applied to populations and situations other than those described in this book. While the model has its origins in children with disruptive behavior disorders, it may also have application to other clinical populations (e.g., youth whose difficulties are along the "internalizing" dimension). This, of course, is an avenue for future exploration. And the degree to which the skills-training component of the CPS model produces verifiable improvements in children's cognitive skills in another area for future examination. Alas, there is more work to be done. Stay tuned.

References

Abidin, R. R. (1995). *Parenting Stress Index professional manual* (3rd ed.). Odessa, FL: Psychological Assessment Resources.

Abikoff, H., & Klein, R. G. (1992). Attention-deficit hyperactivity disorder and conduct disorder: Comorbidity and implications for treatment. *Journal of Consulting and Clinical Psychology, 60,* 881–892.

Akhtar, N., & Bradley, E. J. (1991). Social information processing deficits of aggressive children: Present findings and implications for social skills training. *Clinical Psychology Review, 11,* 621–644.

Alexander, J. F., & Parsons, B. V. (1973). Short-term behavioral intervention with delinquent families: Impact on family process and recidivism. *Journal of Abnormal Psychology, 81,* 219–225.

American Academy of Child and Adolescent Psychiatry. (2002). Practice parameters for the prevention and management of aggressive behavior in child and adolescent psychiatric institutions, with special reference to seclusion and restraint. *Journal of the American Academy of Child and Adolescent Psychiatry, 41*(Suppl.), 4S–25S.

American Psychiatric Association. (1994). *Diagnostic and statistical manual of mental disorders* (4th ed.). Washington, DC: Author.

Amsel, A. (1990). Arousal, suppression, and persistence: Frustration theory, attention, and its disorders. *Cognition and Emotion, 4*(3), 239–268.

Anastopoulos, A. D., Guevremont, D., Shelton, T. L., & DuPaul, G. J. (1992). Parenting stress among families of children with attention deficit hyperactivity disorder. *Journal of Abnormal Child Psychology, 20,* 503–520.

Anderson, K. E., Lytton, H., & Romney, D. M. (1986). Mothers' interactions with normal and conduct-disordered boys: Who affects whom? *Developmental Psychology, 22*, 604–609.

Angold, A., & Costello, E. J. (1993). Depressive comorbidity in children and adolescents: Empirical, theoretical, and methodological issues. *American Journal of Psychiatry, 150*, 1779–1791.

Arnold, E. H., & O'Leary, S. G. (1995). The effect of child negative affect on maternal discipline behavior. *Journal of Abnormal Child Psychology, 23*(5), 585–595.

Atkins, M. S., McKay, M. K., Frazier, S. L., Jacobsons, L. J., Arvantitis, P., Cunningham, T., et al. (2002). Suspensions and detentions in an urban, low-income school: Punishment or reward? *Journal of Abnormal Child Psychology, 30*, 361–372.

Barkley, R. A. (1997a). Behavioral inhibition, sustained attention, and executive functions: Constructing a unifying theory of ADHD. *Psychological Bulletin, 121*(1), 65–94.

Barkley, R. A. (1997b). *Defiant children: A clinician's manual for assessment and parent training* (2nd ed.). New York: Guilford Press.

Barkley, R. A., Anastopoulos, A. D., Guevremont, D., & Fletcher, K. F. (1992). Adolescents with attention-deficit hyperactivity disorder: Mother–adolescent interactions, family beliefs and conflicts, and maternal psychopathology. *Journal of Abnormal Child Psychology, 20*, 263–288.

Baumrind, D. (1968). Authoritarian vs. authoritative parental control. *Adolescence, 3*, 255–272.

Beitchman, J. H., Brownlie, E. B., & Wilson, B. (1996). Linguistic impairment and psychiatric disorders: Pathways to overcome. In J. H. Beitchman, N. J. Cohen, M. M. Konstantareas, & R. Tannock (Eds.), *Language, learning, and behavior disorders: Developmental, biological, and clinical perspectives* (pp. 494–514). New York: Cambridge University Press.

Bell, R. (1968). A reinterpretation of the direction of effects in socialization. *Psychological Review, 75*, 81–95.

Belsky, J. (1980). Child maltreatment: An ecological integration. *American Psychologist, 35*, 320–335.

Belsky, J. (1984). The determinants of parenting: A process model. *Child Development, 55*, 83–96.

Bernal, M. E., Klinnert, M. D., & Schultz, L. A. (1980). Outcome evaluation of behavioral parent training and client-centered parent counseling for children with conduct problems. *Journal of Applied Behavior Analysis, 13*, 677–691.

Beutler, L. (2004). The empirically supported treatments movement: A scientist-practitioner's response. *Clinical Psychology: Science and Practice, 11*(3), 225–229.

Biederman, J., Faraone, S. V., Mick, E., Wozniak, J., Chen, L., Ouellette, C., et al. (1996). Attention-deficit hyperactivity disorder and juvenile mania: An overlooked comorbidity? *Journal of the American Academy of Child and Adolescent Psychiatry, 35*(8), 997–1008.

Biederman, J., Faraone, S. V., Milberger, S., Garcia, J., Chen, L., Mick, E., et al. (1996). Is childhood oppositional defiant disorder a precursor to adolescent conduct disorder?: Findings from a four-year follow-up study of children with ADHD. *Journal of the American Academy of Child and Adolescent Psychiatry, 35*(9), 1193–1204.

Bird, H. R., Gould, M. S., & Staghezza, B. M. (1993). Patterns of diagnostic comorbidity in a community sample of children aged 9 through 16 years. *Journal of the American Academy of Child and Adolescent Psychiatry, 32*(2), 361–368.

Bloomquist, M. L., August, G. J., Cohen, C., Doyle, A., & Everhart, K. (1997). Social problem solving in hyperactive–aggressive children: How and what they think in conditions of controlled processing. *Journal of Clinical Child Psychology, 26*, 172–180.

Borkowski, J. G., & Burke, J. E. (1996). Theories, models, and measurements of executive functioning: An information processing perspective. In G. R. Lyon & N. A. Krasnegor (Eds.), *Attention, memory, and executive function* (pp. 235–262). Baltimore: Brookes.

Brestan, E. V., & Eyberg, S. M. (1998). Effective psychosocial treatment of conduct-disordered children and adolescents: 29 years, 82 studies, and 5,272 kids. *Journal of Clinical Child Psychology, 27*(2), 180–189.

Bretherton, I., Fritz, J., Zahn-Waxler, C., & Ridgeway, D. (1986). Learning to talk about emotions: A functionalist perspective. *Child Development, 57*, 529–548.

Bronowski, J. (1967). Human and animal languages. In T. A. Seboek (Ed.), *To honor Roman Jakobson. Essays on the occasion of his seventieth birthday.* (Vol. 1, pp. 379–394). The Hague, The Netherlands: Mouton.

Bronowski, J. (1976). *The ascent of man.* Cambridge, MA: MIT Press.

Bronowski, J. (1977). *Human and animal languages.* In J. Bronowski (Ed.), *A sense of the future* (pp. 104–131). Cambridge, MA: MIT Press.

Budman, C. L., Bruun, R. D., Park, K. S., & Olson, M. E. (1998). Rage attacks in children and adolescents with Tourette's disorder: A pilot study. *Journal of Clinical Psychiatry, 59*(11), 576–580.

Cantwell, D. P., & Baker, L. (1991). *Psychiatric and developmental disorders in children with communication disorders.* Washington, DC: American Psychiatric Press.

Cavell, T. A. (2000). *Working with parents of aggressive children.* Washington, DC: American Psychological Association.

Chamberlain, P., & Patterson, G. R. (1995). Discipline and child compliance in parenting. In M. H. Bornstein (Ed.), *Handbook of parenting: Vol. 4. Applied and practical parenting* (pp. 205–225). Mahwah, NJ: Erlbaum.

Chambless, D. L., Sanderson, W. C., Shoham, V., Bennett-Johnson, S., Pope, K. S., Crits-Christoph, P., et al. (1996). An update on empirically validated therapies. *Clinical Psychologist, 49*, 5–18.

Charney, R. (2002). *Teaching children to care: Classroom management for ethical and academic growth.* Greenfield, MA: Northeast Foundation for Children.

Chess, S., & Thomas, A. (1984). *Origins and evolution of behavior disorders: From infancy to early adult life.* New York: Brunner/Mazel.

Cicchetti, D., & Lynch, M. (1993). Toward an ecological/transactional model of community violence and child maltreatment. *Psychiatry, 56*, 96–118.

Cicchetti, D., & Lynch, M. (1995). Failures in the expectable environment and their impact on individual development: The case of child maltreatment. In D. Cicchetti & D. J. Cohen (Eds.), *Developmental psychopathology: Vol. 2. Risk, disorder, and adaptation* (pp. 32–71). New York: Wiley.

Cohen, J. (1988). *Statistical power analysis for the behavioral sciences.* New York: Academic Press.

Crockenberg, S., & Litman, C. (1990). Autonomy as competence in two-year-olds: Maternal correlates of child defiance, compliance, and self-assertion. *Developmental Psychology, 26,* 961–971.

Culbertson, J. L., & Willis, D. J. (1992). *Testing young children: A reference guide for developmental, psychoeducational, and psychosocial assessments.* Houston, TX: Pro-Ed.

Davis, A. D., Sanger, D. D., & Morris-Friehe, M. (1991). Language skills of delinquent and nondelinquent adolescent males. *Journal of Communication Disorders, 24,* 251–266.

Denckla, M. B. (1996). A theory and model of executive function: A neuropsychological perspective. In G. R. Lyon & N. A. Krasnegor (Eds.), *Attention, memory, and executive function* (pp. 263–278). Baltimore: Brookes.

Dishion, T. J., French, D. C., & Patterson, G. R. (1995). The development and ecology of antisocial behavior. In D. Cicchetti & D. J. Cohen (Eds.), *Developmental psychopathology: Vol. 2. Risk, disorder, and adaptation* (pp. 421–471). New York: Wiley.

Dishion, T. J., & Patterson, G. R. (1992). Age affects in parent training outcomes. *Behavior Therapy, 23,* 719–729.

Dodge, K. A. (1980). Social cognition and children's aggressive behavior. *Child Development, 51,* 162–170.

Dodge, K. A. (1993). The future of research on the treatment of conduct disorder. *Development and Psychopathology, 5,* 311–319.

Dodge, K. A., & Coie, J. D. (1987). Social information processing factors in reactive and proactive aggression in children's peer groups. *Journal of Personality and Social Psychology, 53,* 1146–1158.

Dodge, K. A., Pettit, G. S., McClaskey, C., & Brown, M. (1986). Social competence in children. *Monographs of the Society for Research in Child Development, 51* (2, Serial No. 213), 213–251.

Dodge, K. A., Price, J. N., Bachorowski, J., & Newman, J. P. (1990). Hostile attributional biases in severely aggressive adolescents. *Journal of Abnormal Psychology, 99,* 385–392.

Douglas, V. I. (1980). High level mental processes in hyperactive children: Implications for training. In R. M. Knights & D. J. Baker (Eds.), *Treatment of hyperactive and learning disordered children: Current research* (pp. 65–92). Baltimore: University Park Press.

Dumas, J. E., & LaFreniere, P. J. (1993). Mother–child relationships as sources of support or stress: A comparison of competent, average, aggressive, and anxious dyads. *Child Development, 64,* 1732–1754.

Dumas, J. E., LaFreniere, P. J., & Serketich, W. J. (1995). "Balance of power": A transactional analysis of control in mother–child dyads involving socially competent, aggressive, and anxious children. *Journal of Abnormal Psychology, 104,* 104–113.

Eslinger, P. J. (1996). Conceptualizing, describing, and measuring components of executive function. In G. R. Lyon & N. A. Krasnegor (Eds.), *Attention, memory, and executive function* (pp. 367–395). Baltimore: Brookes.

Fuster, J. M. (1989). *The prefrontal cortex.* New York: Raven Press.

Fuster, J. M. (1995). Memory and planning: Two temporal perspectives of frontal lobe function. In H. H. Jasper, S. Riggio, & P. S. Goldman-Rakic (Eds.), *Epilepsy and the functional autonomy of the frontal lobe* (pp. 9–18). New York: Raven Press.

Garland, E. J., & Weiss, M. (1996). Case study: Obsessive difficult temperament and its response to serotonergic medication. *Journal of the American Academy of Child and Adolescent Psychiatry, 35*(7), 916–920.

Geller, B., & Luby, J. (1997). Child and adolescent bipolar disorder: Review of the past 10 years. *Journal of the American Academy of Child and Adolescent Psychiatry, 36*(9), 1–9.

Gerard, A. B. (1994). *Parent–Child Relationship Inventory (PCRI) manual.* Los Angeles: Western Psychological Services.

Gilmour, J., Hill, B., Place, M., & Skuse, D. H. (2004). Social communication deficits in conduct disorder: A clinical and community survey. *Journal of Child Psychology and Psychiatry, 45,* 967–978.

Gottlieb, G. (1992). *Individual development and evolution: The genesis of novel behavior.* New York: Oxford University Press.

Gottman, J. (1986). The world of coordinated play: Same and cross-sex friendship in children. In J. M. Gottman & J. G. Parker (Eds.), *Conversations of friends: Speculations on affective development* (pp. 139–191). Cambridge, UK: Cambridge University Press.

Greene, R. W., Biederman, J., Zerwas, S., Monuteaux, M., Goring, J., Faraone, S. V. (2002). Psychiatric comorbidity, family dysfunction, and social impairment in referred youth with oppositional defiant disorder. *American Journal of Psychiatry, 159*(7), 1214–1224.

Greene, R. W. (1996). Students with ADHD and their teachers: Implications of a goodness-of-fit perspective. In T. H. Ollendick & R. J. Prinz (Eds.), *Advances in clinical child psychology* (pp. 205–230). New York: Plenum Press.

Greene, R. W., & Ablon, J. S. (2001). What does the MTA study tell us about effective psychosocial treatment for ADHD? *Journal of Clinical Child Psychology, 30*(1), 114–121.

Greene, R. W., Ablon, J. S., Hassuk, B., Regan, K., Markey, J., Goring, J., & Rabbitt, S. (2005). Elimination of restraint and seclusion and reduction of injuries on an inpatient child psychiatry unit. Manuscript under review.

Greene, R. W., Ablon, J. S., Monuteaux, M., Goring, J., Henin, A., Raezer, L., et al. (2004). Effectiveness of Collaborative Problem Solving in affectively dysregulated youth with oppositional defiant disorder: Initial findings. *Journal of Consulting and Clinical Psychology, 72*(6), 1157–1164.

Greene, R. W., Biederman, J., Faraone, S. V., Sienna, M., & Garcia-Jetton, J. (1997). Adolescent outcome of boys with attention-deficit/hyperactivity disorder and social disability: Results from a 4-year longitudinal follow-up study. *Journal of Consulting and Clinical Psychology, 65*(5), 758–767.

Greene, R. W., Beszterczey, S. K., Katzenstein T., Park, K., & Goring, J. C. (2002). Are students with ADHD more stressful to teach?: Predictors of teacher stress in an elementary-age sample. *Journal of Emotional and Behavioral Disorders, 10,* 79–89.

Hanf, C. (1969, April). *A two-stage program for modifying maternal controlling during mother–child interaction.* Paper presented at the meeting of the Western Psychological Association, Vancouver, British Columbia, Canada.

Harrington, R., Fudge, H., Rutter, M., Pickles, A., & Hill, J. (1991). Adult outcomes of childhood and adolescent depression: II. Links with antisocial disorders. *Journal of the American Academy of Child and Adolescent Psychiatry, 30,* 434–439.

Harter, S. (1983). Developmental perspectives on the self-system. In P. H. Mussen (Series Ed.) & E. M. Hetherington (Vol. Ed.), *Handbook of child psychology, Vol. 4. Socialization, personality, and social development* (pp. 275–385). New York: Wiley.

Hayes, S. C., Gifford, E. V., & Ruckstuhl, L. E. (1996). Relational frame theory and executive function: A behavioral analysis. In G. R. Lyon & N. A. Krasnegor (Eds.), *Attention, memory, and executive function* (pp. 279–306). Baltimore: Brookes.

Hinshaw, S. P. (1992). Intervention for social competence and social skill. *Child and Adolescent Psychiatric Clinics of North America, 1*(2), 539–552.

Hinshaw, S. P., Lahey, B. B., & Hart, E. L. (1993). Issues of taxonomy and comorbidity in the development of conduct disorder. *Development and Psychopathology, 5,* 31–49.

Hoffenaar, P. (2004). *The assessment and development of oppositionality.* Amsterdam, The Netherlands: Print Partners Ipskamp B. V., Enschede.

Hoffman, M. L. (1975). Moral internalization, parental power, and the nature of parent–child interaction. *Developmental Psychology, 11,* 228–239.

Hoffman, M. L. (1983). Affective and cognitive processes in moral internalization. In E. T. Higgins, D. Ruble, & W. Hartup (Eds.), *Social cognition and social development: A sociocultural perspective* (pp. 236–274). New York: Cambridge University Press.

Hollingshead, A. B. (1975). *Four-Factor Index of Social Status.* Unpublished manuscript, Yale University, New Haven, CT.

Ialongo, N. S., Horn, W. F., Pascoe, J. M., Greenberg, G., Packard, T., Lopez, et al. (1993). The effects of a multimodal intervention with attention-deficit hyperactivity disorder children: A 9-month follow-up. *Journal of the American Academy of Child and Adolescent Psychiatry, 32,* 182–189.

Jacobson, N. S., & Truax, P. (1991). Clinical significance: A statistical approach to defining meaningful change in psychotherapy research. *Journal of Consulting and Clinical Psychology, 59,* 12–19.

Kazdin, A. E. (1993). Treatment of conduct disorder: Progress and directions in psychotherapy research. *Development and Psychopathology, 5,* 277–310.

Kazdin, A. E. (1997). Parent management training: Evidence, outcomes, and issues. *Journal of the American Academy of Child and Adolescent Psychiatry, 36*(10), 1349–1356.

Kazdin, A. E., Esveldt-Dawson, K., French, N. H., & Unis, A. S. (1987). Problem-solving skills training and relationship therapy in the treatment of antisocial child behavior. *Journal of Consulting and Clinical Psychology, 55,* 76–85.

Kazdin, A. E., Siegel, T. C., & Bass, D. (1992). Cognitive problem-solving skills training and parent management training in the treatment of antisocial behavior in children. *Journal of Consulting and Clinical Psychology, 60*(5), 733–747.

Kendall, P. C. (1993). Cognitive-behavioral therapies with youth: Guiding theory, current status, and emerging developments. *Journal of Consulting and Clinical Psychology, 61*(2), 235–247.

Kendall, P. C., Chu, B., Gifford, A., Hayes, C., & Nautu, M. (1998). Breathing life into a manual: Flexibility and creativity with manual-based treatments. *Cognitive and Behavioral Practice, 5*, 177–198.

Kendall, P. C., & Southam-Gerow, M. (1995). Issues in the transportability of treatment. *Journal of Consulting and Clinical Psychology, 63*, 702–708.

Kochanska, G. (1993). Toward a synthesis of parental socialization and child temperament in early development of conscience. *Child Development, 64*, 325–347.

Kochanska, G., & Askan, N. (1995). Mother–child mutually positive affect, the quality of child compliance to requests and prohibitions, and maternal control as correlates of early internalization. *Child Development, 66*, 236–254.

Kohn, A. (1996). *Beyond discipline: From compliance to community*. Alexandria, VA: Association for Supervision and Curriculum Development.

Kopp, C. B. (1982). Antecedents of self-regulation: A developmental perspective. *Developmental Psychology, 18*(2), 199–214.

Kopp, C. B. (1989). Regulation of distress and negative emotions: A developmental view. *Developmental Psychology, 25*(3), 343–354.

Lahey, B. B., & Loeber, R. (1994). Framework for a developmental model of oppositional defiant disorder and conduct disorder. In D. K. Routh (Ed.), *Disruptive behavior disorders in childhood* (pp. 139–180). New York: Plenum Press.

Little, S. S. (1993). Nonverbal learning disabilities and socioemotional functioning: A review of recent literature. *Journal of Learning Disabilities, 26*(10), 653–665.

Lochman, J. E., Coie, J. D., Underwood, M. K., & Terry, R. (1993). Effectiveness of a social relations intervention program for aggressive and nonaggressive, rejected children. *Journal of Consulting and Clinical Psychology, 61*(6), 1053–1058.

Lochman, J. E., White, K. J., & Wayland, K. K. (1991). Cognitive-behavioral assessment and treatment with aggressive children. In P.C. Kendall (Ed.), *Child and adolescent therapy: Cognitive-behavioral procedures* (pp. 25–65). New York: Guilford Press.

Loeber, R., & Keenan, K. (1994). Interaction between conduct disorder and its comorbid conditions: Effects of age and gender. *Clinical Psychology Review, 14*(6), 497–523.

Luria, A. R. (1961). *The role of speech in the regulation of normal and abnormal behavior*. New York: Basic Books.

Lyon, G. R. (1996). The need for conceptual and theoretical clarity in the study of attention, memory, and executive function. In G. R. Lyon & N. A. Krasnegor (Eds.), *Attention, memory and executive function* (pp. 3–10). Baltimore: Brookes.

Lytton, H. (1990). Child and parent effects on boys' conduct disorder: A reinterpretation. *Developmental Psychology, 26*, 683–697.

Maccoby, E. E. (1980). *Social development*. New York: Harcourt, Brace, Jovanovich.

McClellan, J. (2005). Commentary: Treatment guidelines for child and adolescent bipolar disorder. *Journal of the American Academy of Child and Adolescent Psychiatry, 44*(3), 236–239.

Milich, R., & Dodge, K. A. (1984). Social information processing in child psychiatric populations. *Journal of Abnormal Child Psychology, 12*, 471–490.

Milner, B. (1995). Aspects of human frontal lobe function. In H. H. Jasper, S. Riggio, & P. S. Goldman-Rakic (Eds.), *Epilepsy and the functional autonomy of the frontal lobe* (pp. 67–81). New York: Raven Press.

Minuchin, S. (1974). *Families and family therapy*. Cambridge, MA: Harvard University Press.

Mischel, W. (1983). Delay of gratification as process and as person variable in development. In D. Magnusson & V. P. Allen (Eds.), *Interactions in human development* (pp. 149–165). New York: Academic Press.

Moffitt, T. E. (1990). The neuropsychology of delinquency: A critical review of theory and research. In N. Morris & M. Tonry (Eds.), *Crime and justice* (Vol. 12, pp. 99–169). Chicago: University of Chicago Press.

Moffitt, T. E., & Henry, B. (1991). Neuropsychological studies of juvenile delinquency and violence: A review. In J. Milner (Ed.), *The neuropsychology of aggression* (pp. 67–91). Norwell, MA: Kluwer Academic.

Moffitt, T. E., & Lynam, D. (1994). The neuropsychology of conduct disorder and delinquency: Implications for understanding antisocial behavior. In D. C. Fowles, P. Sutker, & S. H. Goodman (Eds.), *Experimental personality and psychopathology research 1994* (pp. 233–262). New York: Springer.

Moore, L. A., Hughes, J. N., & Robinson, M. (1992). A comparison of the social information-processing abilities of rejected and accepted hyperactive children. *Journal of Clinical Child Psychology, 21*(2), 123–131.

National Institute of Mental Health. (1985). CGI (Clinical Global Impression Scale). *Psychopharmacological Bulletin, 21*, 839–844.

Ollendick, T. H. (1996). Violence in youth: Where do we go from here? Behavior therapy's response. *Behavior Therapy, 27*, 485–514.

Orvaschel, H. (1994). *Schedule for affective disorders and schizophrenia for school-age children—epidemiologic version*. Ft. Lauderdale, FL: Nova Southeastern University, Center for Psychological Studies.

Patterson, G. R., & Chamberlain, P. (1994). A functional analysis of resistance during parent training therapy. *Clinical Psychology: Science and Practice, 1*(1), 53–70.

Patterson, G. R., DeBaryshe, B.D., & Ramsey, E. (1989). A developmental perspective on antisocial behavior. *American Psychologist, 44*, 329–335.

Patterson, G. R., & Gullion, M.E. (1968). *Living with children: New methods for parents and teachers*. Champaign, IL: Research Press.

Patterson, G. R., Reid, J. B., & Dishion, T. J. (1992). *Antisocial boys*. Patterson, OR: Castalia.

Pelham, W. E., Wheeler, T., & Chronis, A. (1998). Empirically supported treatments for attention-deficit disorder. *Journal of Cinical Child Psychology, 27*(2), 190–205.

Pennington, B. F. (1994). The working memory function of the prefrontal cortices: Implications for developmental and individual differences in cognition. In M. M. Haith, J. Benson, R. Roberts, & B. F. Pennington (Eds.), *The development of future oriented processes* (pp. 243–289). Chicago: University of Chicago Press.

Pennington, B. F., & Ozonoff, S. (1996). Executive functions and developmental psychopathology. *Journal of Child Psychology and Psychiatry, 37*, 51–87.

Perry, D. G., & Perry, L. C. (1983). Social learning, causal attribution, and moral internalization. In C. J. Brainerd (Series Ed.) & J. Bisanz, G.L. Bisanz, & R. Kail (Vol. Eds.), *Learning in children: Progress in cognitive development research* (pp. 105–136). New York: Springer-Verlag.

Piaget, J. (1952). *The origins of intelligence in children*. New York: International Universities Press.

Piaget, J. (1981). *Intelligence and affect: Their relationship during children's development*. Palo Alto, CA: Annual Reviews.

Prinz, R. J., & Miller, G. E. (1994). Family-based treatment for childhood antisocial behavior: Experimental influences on dropout and engagement. *Journal of Consulting and Clinical Psychology, 62*, 645–650.

Quiggle, N. L., Garber, J., Panak, W.F., & Dodge, K.A. (1992). Social information processing in aggressive and depressed children. *Child Development, 63*, 1305–1320.

Rothbart, M. K., & Derryberry, D. (1981). Development of individual differences in temperament. In M. E. Lamb & A. L. Brown (Eds.), *Advances in developmental psychology* (Vol. 1, pp. 37–86). Hillsdale, NJ: Erlbaum.

Rourke, B. P. (1989). *Nonverbal learning disabilities: The syndrome and the model*. New York: Guilford Press.

Rourke, B. P., & Fuerst, D. R. (1995). Cognitive processing, academic achievement, and psychosocial functioning: A neurodevelopmental perspective. In D. Cicchetti & D. J. Cohen (Eds.), *Developmental psychopathology: Vol. 1. Theory and methods* (pp. 391–423). New York: Wiley.

Ryan E. P., Hart, V. S., Messick, D. L., Aaron, J., & Burnette, M. (2004). A prospective study of assault against staff by youths in a state psychiatric hospital. *Psychiatric Services, 55*, 665–670.

Sameroff, A. (1975). Early influences on development: Fact or fancy? *Merrill-Palmer Quarterly, 21*(4), 267–294.

Sameroff, A. (1995). General systems theory and developmental psychopathology. In D. Cicchetti & D.J. Cohen (Eds.), *Developmental psychopathology: Vol. 1. Theory and methods* (pp. 659–695). New York: Wiley.

Sattler, J. M. (1988). *Assessment of children's intelligence* (3rd ed.). San Diego, CA: Author.

Semrud-Clikeman, M., & Hynd, G. W. (1990). Right-hemisphere dysfunction in nonverbal learning disabilities: Social, academic, and adaptive functioning in adults and children. *Psychological Bulletin, 107*(2), 196–209.

Shirk, S. R. (2001). The road to effective child psychological services: Treatment processes and outcome research. In J. N. Hughes & A. M. La Greca (Eds.), *Handbook of psychological services for children and adolescents* (pp. 43–59). London: Oxford University Press.

Snyder, J., Edwards, P., McGraw, K., Kilgore, K., & Holton, A. (1994). Escalation and reinforcement in mother–child conflict: Social processes associated with the development of physical aggression. *Development and Psychopathology, 6*, 305–321.

Stifter, C. A., Spinrad, T. L., & Braungart-Rieker, J. M. (1999). Toward a developmental model of child compliance: The role of emotion regulation in infancy. *Child Development, 70*(1), 21–32.

Stormschak, E., Speltz, M., DeKlyen, M., & Greenberg, M. (1997). Family interactions during clinical intake: A comparison of families of normal or disruptive boys. *Journal of Abnormal Child Psychology, 25*, 345–357.

Taylor, T. K., & Biglan, A. (1998). Behavioral family interventions for improving child rearing: A review of the literature for clinicians and policy makers. *Clinical Child and Family Psychology Review, 1*(1), 41–60.

Vygotsky, L. S. (1987). Thinking and speech. In L. S. Vygotsky & R. W. Rieber (Series Eds.) & A. S. Carton (Vol. Ed.), *The collected works of L. S. Vygotsky: Vol. 1. Problems in general psychology* (pp. 39–285). New York: Plenum Press.

Waschbusch, D. A., Willoughby, M. T., & Pelham, W. E. (1998). Criterion validity and the utility of reactive and proactive aggression: Comparisons to attention deficit hyperactivity disorder, oppositional defiant disorder, conduct disorder, and other measures of functioning. *Journal of Clinical Child Psychology, 27*(4), 396–405.

Webster-Stratton, C. (1984). Randomized trial of two parent-training programs for families with conduct-disordered children. *Journal of Consulting and Clinical Psychology, 52,* 666–678.

Webster-Stratton, C. (1990). Enhancing the effectiveness of self-administered videotape parent training for families with conduct-problem children. *Journal of Abnormal Child Psychology, 18,* 479–492.

Webster-Stratton, C. (1994). Advancing videotape parent training: A comparison study. *Journal of Consulting and Clinical Psychology, 62,* 583–593.

Wechsler, D. (1974). *Manual for the Wechsler Intelligence Scale for Children—Revised.* New York: Psychological Corporation.

Weiner, I. B. (1975). *Principles of psychotherapy.* New York: Wiley.

Wiltz, N. A., & Patterson, G. R. (1974). An evaluation of parent training procedures designed to alter inappropriate aggressive behavior of boys. *Behavior Therapy, 5,* 215–221.

Wozniak, J., & Biederman, J. (1996). A pharmacological approach to the quagmire of comorbidity in juvenile mania. *Journal of Child and Adolescent Psychiatry, 35*(6), 826–828.

Zillman, D. (1988). Cognition–excitation interdependencies in aggressive behavior. *Aggressive Behavior, 14,* 51–64.

Zoccolillo, M. (1992). Co-occurrence of conduct disorder and its adult outcomes with depressive and anxiety disorders: A review. *Journal of the American Academy of Child and Adolescent Psychiatry, 31,* 547–556.

Index